THE

BOTOX BOOK

THE
BOTOX BOOK

MICHAEL A.C. KANE, M.D.

Foreword by Daniel C. Baker, M.D.

ST. MARTIN'S PRESS ᴀ NEW YORK

This book is for informational purposes only. It is not intended to take the place of medical advice from a trained professional. Readers are advised to consult a physician before acting on any of the information in this book. The fact that an organization or physician is listed on the author's Web site as a possible source of advice or treatment does not mean that the publisher endorses those recommendations.

BOTOX® is a registered trademark of Allergan, Inc. This book has not been authorized, sponsored, prepared, or approved by Allergan, Inc., or any affiliated organization.

www.stmartins.com

Book design by Kathryn Parise

ISBN 0-312-31048-X

First Edition: August 2002

10 9 8 7 6 5 4 3 2 1

CONTENTS

AUTHOR'S NOTE

I have served as an advisory board member for Allergan, the parent company that produces and distributes Botox throughout the United States. I have also done work for them, speaking on their behalf at various meetings around the world. As an advisory board member, I helped to devise the curriculum that the company put together to teach new physician injectors how to properly inject Botox. I have also been compensated for teaching physicians directly from this curriculum. I am not an Allergan employee. I have been granted no stock options by the company and am not under contract to them except for my agreement not to disclose proprietary information that I have learned from them as an advisory board member.

I have also served as an advisory board member for Elan, the parent company that produces and distributes Myobloc throughout the United States. I am also not under contract to this company.

Neither company has tried to influence my relationship with the other. Neither company was told about this book until after the contract was signed and the book was written. Neither company has had any influence whatsoever over the content of this book.

ACKNOWLEDGMENTS

First and foremost, my thanks go out to my patients. Many of the patients whose photos appear in this book have been with me since I first started my practice. They trusted me and took a leap of faith with me when I told them that I thought injecting some botulinum toxin into their faces might help them. It is only through their trust that this book and my work with Botox was possible.

As far as physicians go, I must first thank the man who first said the word *Botox* to me. He is my friend Richard Lisman, a fine oculoplastic surgeon whose office is conveniently right across the street from mine. Richard has a sterling reputation as the man who has kept a great many plastic surgeons and nonplastic surgeons out of hot water by beautifully correcting some problematic results.

I have considered Daniel Baker my mentor for a decade. Besides being an outstanding surgeon, and a great teacher of surgery, Dan has given me invaluable advice and guidance, especially during my early years when I decided to open my own practice. If not for Dan's assistance, I don't know if I would have survived those early dog-eat-dog years as a solo young plastic surgeon in Manhattan.

Sherrell J. Aston has been my department chairman and friend for a decade. Early in the lean years of my practice, he allowed me to assist him in the operating room and actually paid me for it. I would have done it for free. He also gave me my "big break" by allowing me, then a relative unknown, to speak on Botox injections at the Manhattan Eye, Ear and Throat meeting back in 1996. After this initial twenty-minute lecture, I was on the speaker circuit for good.

William B. Nolan was my program director when I was a fellow at the Manhattan Eye, Ear and Throat Hospital. It was under his guidance that I first began doing Botox injections.

When I first began to perform Myobloc injections in 1991, I was greatly aided by Corey Maas. Corey probably has injected the largest number of patients with Myobloc for cosmetic purposes.

But not all the doctors I have to acknowledge are plastic surgeons. I want to thank Arnie Klein of Beverly Hills for being an incredibly honest speaker. Arnie always attributes new things that he has heard to the person who actually said them. Sadly, this is not a very common practice. I also want to thank him for teaching me how to skillfully inject collagen in layers so that my patients' lips turn out full but natural-looking. And I want to thank Fred Brandt of Miami, and now also Manhattan, for his grace when we have disagreed over a few small points in the past. To many physicians, that crime leaves you no longer on speaking terms. Fred, I hope you've learned as much from me as I've learned from you.

A special thanks goes out to my sisters, Kathleen and Karen, who, whenever I had an idea or new area to inject were always willing volunteers who let their slightly mad younger brother try something different on them.

Other physicians, laypeople, office staff, and friends who have helped me tremendously include, in no particular order: Issa, Tracy, CHS, Jo Jo, J. P., Skinny, Snoot, Jordan, Cathy, Olga, Marielle, Joan Kron, Meredith Bernstein, RDM, Dana, Lad, Mickey, and of course Buck.

FOREWORD

~~~~~~
~~~~~~

It's been over a decade since I first met Michael Kane in the halls of the Manhattan Eye, Ear and Throat Hospital. He was an aesthetic surgery fellow and I was his attending surgeon, so we developed a close relationship over the years.

In the years since we met, I would say that Mike has become one of the world's leading experts on botulinum toxin, more commonly known as Botox, and certainly one of the most knowledgeable doctors in the country on this topic. He travels the globe lecturing about Botox and teaching other physicians how to use the substance correctly and creatively. His presentations are always informative, refreshing, and honest. He has superb aesthetic judgment and technical ability.

He also has terrific timing. I had known that he was working on a book about Botox for some time. Now that Botox has been approved by the Food and Drug Administration to treat frown lines, there has never been a greater demand for information on the subject. Even before the media frenzy surrounding the drug's FDA approval, Botox had become the most popular cosmetic technique in the United States.

It's important to remember that with all surgical procedures, the success of the treatment is entirely dependent on the skill of the surgeon.

With Botox, the results are entirely injector-dependent. Proper dosage and proper placement are crucial to the success of the treatment. You want to make sure that the physician disseminating this information is a person with expertise and experience. Mike is the best man for this job. He's very articulate and practical in his presentation, and his aesthetic sense is unmatched. He's also an innovator, extending the uses of Botox throughout all areas of the face, and even the neck. And he has explored the possibilities of the neurotoxin beyond the realm of cosmetic surgery, treating patients with paralysis to even out the movements of the face. He's soft spoken and very low key, not the most common qualities in the cosmetic surgery community. Because of his demeanor and obvious ability, he comes across as a very forthright and ethical physician. He's highly selective about whom he treats in his own practice. And I believe in what he does so completely that I have put a great deal of trust in him to care for my patients when I'm traveling or unavailable. To me, this is the highest compliment I can pay. Please enjoy *The Botox Book*, and know that it was written by capable hands.

—DANIEL C. BAKER, M.D.

HOW TO READ THIS BOOK

I don't want to get off on the wrong foot with you. And, I realize that this is a rather obnoxious title for a chapter of a book. But I didn't know what else to call it and still somehow convince you, the reader, to read it. When I see a preface or acknowledgments in the table of contents followed by Roman numerals (indicating that they aren't really pages at all) I think I skim through it maybe about 10 percent of the time. But you shouldn't skip or skim this chapter. Not because my writing is so inspiring or because every sentence contains such an incredible epiphany that your life would be diminished if each word were not carefully read. But because if you don't read it, you might not really know how to take the rest of the book. While it may be a shame that I've skipped some prefaces in books that I've read, I don't feel that I've misunderstood the books that followed. With this book, misunderstanding is a real possibility. I feel that it is absolutely necessary that the reader read this section, because I will now tell you what this book is and what it is not.

This book is is an explanation of my past experiences using Botox injections to help thousands of patients improve their appearance. It is a book that I hope conveys my utter enthusiasm for the great things that

Botox can do for most of us, and the things that it may do for us in the future. It is a frank book, which will also detail some of the unwanted effects of Botox injections gone awry. It is a book that will show you some things Botox can do that you were not aware of before.

What this book is not is a guarantee of anyone's results. It is absolutely not a replacement for careful consideration, examination, and consultation with your physician with regard to your face and neck and how Botox may help you. It is not a textbook. It is not a book filled with long scientific words that you won't be able to pronounce or understand.

It is also not a book that every doctor actively injecting Botox will agree with. With Botox injections, as with most of the aesthetic procedures available to improve one's looks, there is quite a bit of disagreement. Not every injector—even injectors that I have the utmost respect for—will agree with everything in this book. This book represents my point of view, which has been shaped over eleven years, thousands of injections, and an almost obsessive review of the scientific literature. It has been said that even regular, good old ordinary medicine is both an art and a science. If that is the case, aesthetic procedures are probably two-thirds art and one-third science. Just try to get two artists to decide on whose art is more correct. I'm not pompous enough to call myself an artist, but I do think anyone involved in anesthetics should at least be an artisan or a careful craftsman. I know that some passages in this book will be controversial in the medical community. Where this is the case, I have included photographs to help illustrate my point.

While this book is based on science, it is not a textbook or reference book. Science and anatomy are the basis for what is presented in these pages. But once you get past these initial basics, this book deals with craftsmanship in using this science to improve one's appearance. For that reason, there are no footnotes or copious references to scientific papers and presentations that have already been made public. Many photos have been included to help illustrate the points in the various chapters. It may be a pain in the neck to flip back and forth between the text pages and color photos, but I think that your understanding and appreciation for the content of this book will be increased if you do so. The photos have been chosen to illustrate key points from the text. While I feel it is very important at a scientific meeting to see Botox photos taken before and after injection, with the patient both in full animation and repose, that is not necessary for the layperson. These photos have not been altered in any way to improve the results. There is no trick photography in these pages.

I am not a psychiatrist, I am a plastic surgeon. That said, psychiatry is a large part of plastic surgery: The entire point of improving a patient's appearance is to make that person feel better about himself or herself. These pages contain many comments, personal thoughts, and biases. Some of them have to do with insights into patients' motivation and happiness.

While the photos are not repetitive, some portions of the text may be, so that if readers want to jump ahead to a certain chapter, they should be able to understand it without backtracking. Obviously, it would be best if you started at the beginning and went straight through to the end. But I know that is not how every reader approaches this kind of book. If you start from the beginning, thank you for bearing with the occasional repetitive sentence in subsequent chapters.

Just as this book can be read either by jumping around or from start to finish, the photos can be used in two ways as well. The text in the chapters goes over the photos, and what they illustrate, in detail. It will truly help you to understand what Botox can do for an average patient. However, if you're someone who likes to jump straight to the pictures, there are short captions included that will guide you through the main points illustrated.

Who Should Read this Book

Although everyone is a bit different, there are a few archetypes that most of my patients fit into. Some of these archetypes are included below.

NO, NOT ME, NEVER

In this book, you'll meet people like Claire, a mother of three and grandmother of two. Now in her sixties, she recently went back to work. She has never been one to obsess about appearances. She dresses well but doesn't really care if her look is considered stylish. She hasn't changed her hair in twenty years and likes it the way it is. What she doesn't like is her reflection the mirror. Not that she's fighting the aging process tooth and nail. Far from it. Her medicine cabinet is filled with lotions, toners, exfoliants, and cleansers that she rarely uses—the result of the occasional Mother's Day gift box of over-the-counter skin care lines from the local department store. But it annoys her that her outward appearance doesn't match how great she feels inside.

Claire was reluctant to visit a doctor about her appearance. She didn't see the point of it, since she could never imagine herself having plastic surgery. Neither Claire nor anyone in her family or circle of friends has ever had any plastic surgery. When she finally made an appointment, she insisted she didn't want to discuss anything that involved cutting or stitching. Spending an extra fifteen minutes every morning and evening to properly apply various lotions and potions just wasn't her style either.

Claire had never heard of Botox. But fifteen minutes in the doctor's office every four or five months turned out to be just the thing for her, once she had all the facts. And now when Claire catches a glimpse of herself reflected in a store window, she's pleased with what she sees. Finally, it seems to her, she looks like her true self again.

THE TRENDSETTER

Kathy started from a much different place. She's in her fifties, with two grown children, and delights in attending several formal charity events each year, always wearing the newest look of the season. She will proudly tell anyone who asks (and many who don't) that she had her eyes "done" for her fortieth birthday, and her face lifted eight years later. She sees a very expensive dermatologist—he's quoted in all the magazines—and has been getting Botox injections in her forehead for four years now.

Kathy is happy with how those areas look, but what bothers her now are the little lines coming down from the corners of her mouth, the dimples she sees in her chin when she's having an animated conversation, and the two cords that seem to be running from her chin down her neck. But her dermatologist told her Botox is good only for the upper third of the face—and sold her $300 worth of skin care products. Her plastic surgeon recommended another facelift for the cords in her neck, but said even that wouldn't help with her chin or the lines above it. In any event, Kathy didn't want to go through that painful process all over again so soon.

So she sought out further advice and eventually learned that Botox was just the solution she needed—but only in properly trained hands. Within weeks she got injections from a new practitioner experienced in more than the routine upper third of the face. At the next ball, in another smashing new outfit, she felt fully satisfied with her look, chin, neck, and all.

OVERWORKED AND UNDERAPPRECIATED

And then there's Karen, a working mom in her forties. Karen works at an advertising agency and her days are jam-packed from dawn until the kids fall asleep at night. She feels run down and ragged, and barely has any time for herself—and she knows she looks it. There are a few very ambitious younger workers at her firm, and Karen suspects that her slightly more distinguished appearance may be hurting her position in the company and keeping her from a raise that she knows she deserves.

She wishes there were something she could do to help her appearance now but doesn't relish the prospect of plastic surgery. What she's heard about Botox is that it is the deadly botulism poison, could paralyze her face, and make her look very unnatural. It seems like mainly a celebrity thing, anyway—she doesn't know anyone who has had it.

So when Karen finally made a doctor's appointment to discuss her options, she was surprised by the facts she learned about Botox. Once she knew the truth, it seemed to be the exact solution she was looking for. It wasn't long before she had her first injections. And not much longer after that her raise came through—with a promotion. She'll never know for sure, but in her heart of hearts, Karen thinks looking younger gave her a well-timed boost at the office.

THE THINKER

But Botox isn't a "ladies only" club. Ted, in his forties, divorced, and recently transitioned into a new job, has never been one to stare in the mirror. He considers himself a man's man. He works for a company that provides bartenders, waiters, and waitresses for large affairs. He is the executive in charge of training. His job is to get his employees in a hospitality frame of mind. He insists that all of his people smile while addressing a guest. There's just one problem: Ted has a permanent frown line between his eyebrows, which has been there since his early thirties. Even in the best of moods, he appears to be scowling. That isn't, to say the least, good for his employees or the guests—or his dates, for that matter.

Ted has heard a little bit about Botox and secretly wonders if it might be right for him. But is it only for starlets? Is it safe? Is it expensive? He's not sure, and it isn't as if he can ask his friends about it. And he hasn't seen a doctor since that time he had to go to the ER for stitches eight years ago.

Botox is also not for everyone. There are a few rare medical conditions and some medications that do not mix well with Botox. These and other prohibitions are listed on pages 21 and 111.

Read the Label

You may have heard a little bit about Botox over the past few years, but unless you have been living in a cave, you have heard a lot about it since April 15, 2002. No, not because the IRS said it was a deductible business expense (which it should be, according to people in sales who have had it) but because that is the day that its FDA approval came through. Before then, all cosmetic use of Botox was off-label. What you are probably unaware of is that for most patients who get it done, its use is still off-label.

So what exactly does off-label mean? Basically, when the FDA evaluates a drug, it wants studies that show the drug is safe and effective for a particular purpose. The cosmetic FDA approval for Botox was limited to the frowning area between the eyes for patients sixty-five and under. Does that mean it does *not* work for people over sixty-five? No. Does that mean it does *not* work in the forehead? No. What it means is that the FDA was not provided with enough data yet to rule it is safe and effective in these cases. Does that mean that the FDA thinks that it is unsafe? No. Each use for a medication needs years of studies to prove that it is safe and effective. This is a very expensive and lengthy process. Not every company bothers to go through this process for every use for every drug. So is it illegal to use a drug for a nonapproved purpose? No, this is termed off-label use. Basically, off-label use means finding a new use for a drug that was already found to be safe and effective for another purpose. Aspirin was used as a preventative clot-buster in cardiac patients for many years before the FDA approved it for this use. This off-label use conservatively saved thousands of lives. A company cannot advertise a drug for off-label use, which is why some of you have not heard much about Botox until after April 15, 2002.

THE
BOTOX BOOK

1

THE BUZZ ON BOTOX

A Brief History of Botox

Botox is nothing short of a major breakthrough in fighting the aging process. Safe, effective, noninvasive yet long-lasting (but not irreversible), Botox injections have revolutionized how and why we stay looking and feeling young.

Botox may be news to you, but it has actually been used for a variety of medical reasons since the 1970s. A pediatric ophthalmologist named Dr. Alan Scott pioneered working with the drug, using it for various problems relating to the eyes. His first publication concerning botulinum toxin A (the trade name Botox was not born yet) was published in 1973, detailing his work with rhesus monkeys. Using this powerful new drug to help humans started shortly thereafter. Perhaps Scott's most successful application was for patients with strabismus, or "crossed eyes." When a patient is cross-eyed, one of the six small muscles that move the eye in the socket is weak. Botox is used to weaken the opposing muscle, bringing the eye into alignment. Later, Botox was also used for spasms of the muscles in the eyelid and other muscle spasms throughout the face and neck. But for a long time, Botox was nearly unknown outside the field of ophthalmology.

In 1991, while I was a fellow at the Manhattan Eye, Ear and Throat Hospital, I coauthored a paper with Dr. Richard Lisman, an ophthalmologist, Dr. William Nolan, my program director, and Dr. Thomas Rees, the chairman of the plastic surgery department. In the medical world, a "paper" is either a presentation at a peer review meeting or a publication about a new idea or way to do things in a peer-reviewed journal. Frequently, a paper is both. This paper was presented in 1992 and published in 1998. It had to do with a relatively new method of removing bags from the lower eyelid by using an incision inside the eyelid. I worked very closely with Dr. Lisman on this paper. We became quite friendly, and in the course of our work, we had many discussions outside the scope of our paper. One day, when the paper was nearly finished, Dr. Lisman and I were trying to think of ideas for a new paper. We were discussing what was relatively new in the fields of plastic surgery and ophthalmology. I mentioned to him the new deep chemical peels that plastic surgeons were using to smooth wrinkles from the skin, and he mentioned the word *Botox* to me for the first time. He said it was being used to correct muscle spasms around the eye. I asked him how Botox worked, and he explained it was a substance that, when injected into a muscle, would paralyze it temporarily.

At just that time, I was caring for a patient who was contemplating surgery. She was planning to have a coronal browlift—an operation to eliminate the frown lines on her forehead. This involved making an incision from one ear to the other across the top of her head, and folding the front part of her hair and her entire forehead down across the rest of her face, so that I could surgically remove the muscles between her eyebrows responsible for frowning, and throw them away. After this sort of procedure, there is no going back!

This patient was relatively young and had no other problems. Her eyebrows were not very low and did not need to be raised. She had worn bangs through most of her adult life just to attempt to cover the lines on her forehead, and she was sick of it. She was so irritated by these lines that she was going to have a two-hour operation, requiring general anesthesia (with all its attendant hazards), and necessitating a two-week recovery. I thought I had a better idea.

I went to the medical library and read everything I could find on Botox, carefully researching its effects, mechanism of action, dosage, and side effects. Despite the fact that no one had yet written a paper describing its use for cosmetic purposes, a great deal of information was available about the medication. Its use in the world of ophthalmology had been extensively described and the muscles it had been used on in this arena were similar in size to the muscles that I first wanted to inject. Another muscle that I thought would be a good candidate for injection (the muscle that causes crow's feet) had already been injected for medical purposes, because in some people this muscle goes into a severe spasm, nearly closing the eye. I figured I'd wait and see what kind of result my first patient had with only the frowning muscles injected. Baby steps. The other reason that so much information was available was that botulism was still a significant health hazard in the third world and so a great deal of research funding was directed toward both the botulism bacteria and the eight different types of chemicals it secreted.

When I was satisfied, I drew up my plans, discussed them with Dr. Lisman and Dr. Nolan, and, with their approval, broached the subject with my patient. I had to explain, of course, that this was something that had not been done before but that the medication itself had been injected into many patients for other reasons over more than a decade with an excellent safety record. When my patient agreed to try it out, I borrowed some Botox from the eye department and injected her. It took about two minutes.

Three days later, after essentially no recovery period, no downtime, no swelling, and no bruising, the result was even better than I had dared hope. Where this patient once had deep, irregular frown lines and a seemingly constant scowl, she now had smoother skin and a pleasant countenance. Her frown lines were gone, and a revolution in aesthetic procedures had begun.

From that point on, I quickly expanded the applications of Botox to the entire face and neck, and demonstrated that wherever there are wrinkles that are at least partially caused by muscles, Botox can be effective.

I don't want you to think I was some sort of mad scientist. I didn't dive into this without consulting my superiors. Research was done, papers were read. The leap between hearing how Botox worked and envisioning its working cosmetically throughout the face and neck was not so great as it may seem at first glance. It was very logical. I was already a fully trained plastic surgeon with seven years of working 100 to 110 hours per week under my belt. Rather than enter practice, I decided to pursue a fellowship in aesthetic plastic surgery. This would be an additional year of training. But I didn't do just any fellowship. At that time, the Manhattan Eye, Ear and Throat Hospital fellowship was the holy grail of plastic surgical training. I would operate all day long with the biggest names in plastic surgery. Fellows had their own clinics where patients would flock for me to do their facelifts, liposuction, rhinoplasties, and so forth under the watchful eye of one of my senior surgeons. To this day, the Manhattan Eye, Ear and Throat Hospital performs more cosmetic plastic surgery operations than any other hospital in the world.

It was here that I met Dr. Daniel Baker. Many people recognize that name as belonging to one of the great cosmetic plastic surgeons, but Dan is also perhaps the world's expert in the treatment of facial paralysis. I was fortunate to assist him during several operations to resuspend the paralyzed side of a patient's face. The appearance of someone who has one side of his or her face paralyzed is quite strange. One side looks completely different from the other, yet you can tell they both belong to the same person. The paralyzed side droops, sags, and looks much worse overall than the normal side. During surgical correction, the weak side is elevated and sometimes muscles are redirected to make the face more symmetric. The procedure is akin to a one-sided facelift, browlift, and eyelid tuck. But there is something undeniably paradoxical about the appearance of the paralyzed side. While that side of the face looks worse overall, in small snippets it looks much younger. Sure, the neck is sagging more on that side and the eyebrow is way too low, but the forehead is smooth as glass. The eyes look odd because the lower eyelid is sagging, but there are no crow's feet. The cheek almost appears to be sliding off the face, but there is no smile line on that side. I often thought how perfect it would be if we could get enough strength and lift back into the damaged side but not enough so that it would age like the "good" side.

The other reason I thought Botox would work in many areas of the face was that already several papers had been published describing procedures that rejuvenate the face by weakening it. I thought Botox could be the perfect balancing act. It would allow most of the muscles to work at full strength, but might be precise enough that I could weaken just those muscles or parts of muscles that prematurely age the face. None of this had yet been described in the medical literature, so I started counting the patients I treated. I had injected several dozen patients by 1992 and began to prepare my technique for publication. I wanted to include at least fifty patients to give my study heft. In those early days, patients willing to undergo this treatment were few and far between. I was new in practice—and looked it. Even patients who called to make an appointment based on how their friends appeared after I injected them were skeptical. They would look at me as though I were crazy when I told them exactly what I proposed injecting into their faces. Despite what I told them about the safety and prior experience with this drug, only about one out of four patients I discussed this with went through with the injection. Unfortunately, in the end that meant I was beaten to the publication punch in 1992 by the Carruthers, a husband and wife ophthalmologist/dermatologist team who published the first description of Botox usage for cosmetic reasons, which detailed the effects in eighteen patients.

From there, the field of Botox advanced rapidly. In the mid-'90s, I presented my work and experience with Botox injections throughout the face and neck to approximately fifteen hundred plastic surgeons, only a handful of whom had even heard of Botox, let alone used it. Five short years later, Botox injections were the single most common aesthetic procedure performed in the United States. In 2001, there were 1.6 million

Botox injections performed in the United States alone. The strikingly good results, extremely low risk of complications, lack of any downtime, and ease of procedure have combined to make Botox the beauty world's hottest commodity.

The Truth About Botox

Over the last three to four years, there have been many magazine and newspaper articles about Botox. Yet a lack of decent information remains a problem. No one magazine article can do justice to a substance with so many uses. Another reason is the slant occasionally given to Botox articles. Some writers' primary purpose when writing a piece seems to be entertainment. Writing about frozen faces, Dorian Gray, and a world of expressionless Stepford wives no doubt grabs readers more easily than medical terminology describing cause and effect.

As Botox becomes more and more popular, more articles are being written about it. Unfortunately, many of the "experts" quoted in articles are not experts at all but rather doctors with good PR representation and press contacts. Since the FDA approval was given on April 15, 2002, it seems as though every time certain doctors describe when they began using Botox, the year inches backward in time. Very often the "experts" know little more than the writer writing the story. Shortly before FDA approval, there was an article in the *New York Times* in which, in my opinion, at least half the information given by the physicians was inaccurate or at least not in step with the latest studies and medical reports. This book will set the record straight. Starting with:

Botox Is Not Botulism

One of trickiest tasks with my earliest Botox patients during the early '90s was explaining clearly that I would be not be giving them botulism with their injections. Even now, occasionally a patient will think that the two are equivalent. With the recent meteoric rise of Botox injections and the many magazine articles and news snippets devoted to them, this impression is finally fading. I want to put it to rest once and for all, so that no more patients need to harbor a vague fear in the back of their minds.

One of the things that made my early patients so reluctant to have Botox injections was the fact that most of them remembered that there was an outbreak of botulism in certain canned foods in the United States in the early '70s. And the fact is, botulism remains a serious health hazard across the world. In the United States, there are still sporadic cases of botulism every year, usually attributed to improperly home-canned food in adults and honey ingestion in infants. However, botulism and Botox are not the same thing.

There are many different forms of the disease commonly known as botulism. According to *Internal Medicine* (fifth edition), the most common form of botulism in the United States occurs when a person ingests food contaminated with the botulism bacteria. This bacteria is named *Clostridium botulinum.* When someone eats food containing the bacteria, the bacteria makes itself right at home in the stomach and intestines and begins multiplying. That's when the infected person begins to feel ill.

Each botulinum bacteria infecting the patient secretes a small amount of a chemical—the botulinum toxin. Because the person is now infected with a huge number of bacteria, however, the amount of toxin overall is not small. And since the bacteria are living in the sick person's intestines, the chemical goes directly into the bloodstream and is distributed throughout all the muscles of the body. It is now in the bloodstream and in every muscle of the body in large quantities, and all of the body's muscles become paralyzed. The final way that botulism kills a victim is by paralyzing the muscles normally used to breathe: the patient literally suffocates.

Here is the key part: what is in a Botox injection is a minuscule amount of the chemical secreted by the botulism bacteria. There is absolutely no bacteria—nothing alive—in the Botox injection. A Botox injection does not give you an infection. What it does give you is a very small amount of the chemical, injected precisely into selected muscles to weaken them. Several different types of the chemical have been identified. Botox is a preparation of botulinum toxin A.

How Botox Works

Botox is injected into a muscle to produce a paralyzing effect, but it doesn't actually do anything directly to the muscle itself. Its entire effect is, rather, on the nerves. For a muscle to work it needs a signal. That signal starts in the brain, and goes down the spinal cord and out through the nerves. At the end of the nerve there is a connection to the muscle across a small gap. For the nerve to tell the muscle to work, a small amount of a chemical is released from the end of the nerve. That chemical crosses the gap and causes the muscle to move.

Botox prevents the release of this chemical. Nothing is released to cross the gap and tell the muscle to move. Without the nerve to tell the muscle to move, that small part of the muscle is paralyzed. Most muscles have many thousands of nerve endings that tell them to move. Each nerve ending controls only a small amount of the muscle. However, since the muscle itself is unaltered, if you were to give the muscle a small stimulation or electric shock directly, it would move. The muscle remains in fine working order. Botox only prevents the nerve from telling the muscle to move.

While we're on the subject of nerves, let me clear up another misconception about Botox. It does not cause numbness. There are two different sets of nerves in the body. One set, the sensory nerves, gives us feeling through the skin. Another, very different set of nerves, tells muscles to move. Botox only affects the nerves that control muscles. It does not affect the sensory nerves. Botox does not—*cannot*—make your skin numb.

The effects of Botox are temporary. Once Botox has bound to a nerve, that nerve ending stops being able to tell its part of the muscle to move.

When this happens, that nerve begins to branch out to send a new nerve ending to the muscle to tell it to move. When it is eventually successful in its new growth, the nerve-muscle connection is reestablished and the signals for the muscle to move get through again. This reconnection usually takes about ten to twelve weeks to occur. New data also shows that the original nerve ending may also recover and begin telling that muscle what to do. While this may happen, researchers think that a new connection is the initial pathway to recovery for the muscle.

However, just because the muscle can move doesn't mean that it can move at full strength. Think about what happens if you break your arm and have to wear a cast for three months. When the cast is removed, you are able to move your arm, but very weakly. You need months of physical therapy before that arm is close to the strength of your other arm again. The same thing happens with Botox. Just because you begin to move your muscles after about three months doesn't mean that muscle function is back to full strength. It will probably take *another* three or four months before your muscles come back to full strength—along with your wrinkles.

So when I am asked (as I very often am) how long Botox injections last, I generally say that in most areas, you can expect excellent results for about three months, with somewhat diminishing returns for an additional three months. Some patients do not want any additional movement and come in regularly at three months or at the first sign of movement. Some patients wait about six or seven months, until all of the effect is gone. On average, though, I see most patients every four to five months when they first start out with injections. The longer their course of treatment, however, the less frequently they need them.

Another common question patients have is how much the injections will hurt. Any injection, even one done with a needle as small as the one used for Botox injections, can cause some pain. With a needle this small, the pinprick pain is minimal. What does hurt a bit is the fact that when done properly, Botox injections are into the muscle. If you have ever had a tetanus shot in your rear end or shoulder, you know what I mean. Icing the area before the procedure keeps this pain to a minimum.

If you do feel a bit traumatized after your first injection, hang in there. Nearly every patient says the first injection is the roughest.

The Old, the Young, and the New

Botox was initially used and then received its FDA approval for muscular spasms around the face and neck. As you will soon find out, it has myriad cosmetic uses throughout the face and neck. I have also used it in the chest, forearms, and hands. And there are literally hundreds of non-cosmetic, medicinal uses for Botox that have been published in the scientific literature.

There is a reason there are hundreds of uses for Botox and only one for most other medications. While many medicines have been developed to have a very specific action, Botox has a very basic action. Botox stops a nerve from communicating with a muscle. This is a rudimentary interaction that occurs in thousands of ailments. For this reason, the possibilities for Botox use in the future are limitless.

The Poison Pen

Is Botox a poison or not? To my way of thinking, it's all a question of degree. If you were writing a murder mystery would it make sense to have your protagonist do in his victim with some Botox-laced food or drink? Yes, if your murderer were a fictional Bill Gates. There is so little Botox in one very expensive vial that doing away with someone in this manner would be prohibitively expensive for most of us.

Aspirin has a lot in common with Botox, for example. It too has a very basic action. It stops the platelets in your blood from performing some of their tasks. Since hundreds of reactions throughout the body are mediated by platelets, aspirin has many uses. In fact, it is probably the most widely used drug in the world. One aspirin a day may help a cardiac patient to live longer. Two may make your headache better or bring down a dangerously high fever. Take the whole bottle and you will not wake up. With Botox—as with many widely used drugs—a little can be very good for you while a lot will kill you.

2

WHO BENEFITS FROM BOTOX?

Slackers and Scowlers from Twenty-plus and Up

Many patients have misconceptions about the appropriate age to use Botox. Some younger patients believe that only older people with many lines on their faces can benefit from Botox. Some older patients believe that since they have thinned, excess, or hanging skin, Botox can't help them, and that it only truly works in younger patients.

Actually, Botox is one of the few rejuvenative treatments that can benefit patients of almost any age. Most of the patients who can profit from Botox injections are in their early thirties or above. However, I have injected many people in their twenties. Some of these young patients have facial habits that predispose them to develop deep frown or worry lines very early in life. These patients often frown or raise their eyebrows for emphasis when talking to people, not just to indicate anger or surprise as most people do. Due to this facial behavior pattern, they develop lines and wrinkles on their faces literally decades before their contemporaries. I should know, I was one of them. Early in my practice, my schoolteacher sister would work in my office for one week during each summer so I could give my receptionist a week off. After the end of one long day in which I had injected one patient after another with Botox, my sister cornered me. She thought it was ridiculous that I was recommending and performing these injections on patients when my brow was in worse shape than many of theirs. I looked in the mirror and had to admit she was right. I was only thirty but I had a habit of frowning when speaking as a way to emphasize my point. I had also developed another very bad habit.

During a Botox consultation, the patient is asked to make several different facial expressions followed by a relaxed face. Typically, the exam goes something like this: Please frown, relax, frown again, harder, relax, smile, relax, smile harder, relax, squint, relax, raise your eyebrows, relax, show me your lower teeth, relax, and so on. I'm not exactly sure why but very often the patient will have a hard time making the expression requested. Some patients also raise their eyebrows when I ask them to frown. They are probably a little nervous, and some patients find it hard to make these expressions without looking in a mirror. To help them along, I found myself contorting my own face along with my instructions. So my face was being scrunched into severe line-forming mode hundreds of times a day in addition to my usual animation. I was also what I call a frowning concentrator. When I was concentrating while reading, operating, or speaking to others, a sharp frown was always visible across my brow. One injection in the mirror and I became a lot less angry-looking. But not completely at peace. My frown line was so severe that it did not vanish entirely. That took a year or two of rest, courtesy of my Botox injections.

Often, this prematurely aging facial pattern of behavior can be broken with only one or two Botox injections (which was the case with me). Sometimes, this pattern is so ingrained that it is difficult to break the cycle and the patient will need repeated maintenance injections of Botox. Patients in their twenties might also get Botox to avoid a nose job: injecting Botox in the muscles between the nose and lip can eliminate the appearance of a hooked nose. There are muscles that run from the bottom of the nose into the upper lip. When you smile, these muscles contract. While they help to pull your lip up very slightly, they mostly pull the tip of your nose down. This explains why some of you may have thought you looked a little strange in a photo someone took at a party when you weren't looking. You may have thought, "I don't look like that. I don't have a hooked nose." Well you may, sometimes. Most people don't really have a good image in their heads of what they look like in a true profile shot. We can't get that view from a mirror, which provides only a three-quarter view at best. Also, when people look at themselves in a mirror, they tend to unconsciously tilt and turn their heads just so to find the most pleasing image possible. Sorry to say, this is not how other people see us. This is especially true when one is smiling. In the mirror, a smile is always just so. No mini smiles, no tonsil-revealing wide-open guffaw smiles, and no gummy smiles. Just how-we-want-to-look smiles. So when you add up the big smile, the bad angle, the pulling down of the tip of your nose, and throw in the true profile view, the real picture can be disconcerting. Botox can eliminate that smiling pull-down of your nasal tip. Botoxing these muscles won't affect your appearance at rest, just when smiling. And this will pay dividends over the years. Frequently, older patients will undergo rhinoplasty despite the fact that they have been happy with their nose all their life. But after many years of both gravity and these muscles pulling down on the tip of their nose, their nose doesn't look like it used to and it needs to be lifted back up. Botox can help to prevent the aging droopy nose.

Botox is also useful in the younger patient who has had problems with previous chin implant surgery. During chin augmentation an implant, usually made of rubberized silicone, is placed in a pocket directly on top of the jawbone. Usually this is done through an incision just under the chin but sometimes it is inserted via an incision in the mouth between the lower gums and lower lip. When the pocket is made, the muscles of the chin are detached from the bone to create space for the implant. Rarely, this can result in unusual dimples and wrinkling of the chin during normal everyday facial expressions. This unwanted effect is often even more pronounced if the chin implant is removed. In this case, the muscles reattach themselves to the bone but sometimes in not exactly the right place, leading to severe wrinkling and dimpling of the chin especially when the lips are closed tightly. Botox is very effective in eliminating these wrinkles when injected very carefully. The chin muscles are attached by strong fibers to the undersurface of the skin of the chin. When the muscles contort, this strange pattern is transmitted to the chin, making it visible on the face. The key to injecting this area is that only the superficial part of the muscle should be weakened with Botox. This will smooth out the wrinkles of the skin but leave the deep portion of the muscles strong so that normal movement, including closing the lips, is maintained.

The above examples illustrate an important point about Botox. In my mind, the primary benefit of Botox is to help patients look *better,* not necessarily *younger.* Very often Botox does help patients appear more youthful. But patients in their twenties are not trying to look younger, just better.

Most patients, though, are in their thirties and older and use Botox to help eliminate premature signs of aging and wrinkling throughout the face. This is the most remarkable thing about Botox: it is truly a preventative procedure against aging. There are many treatments out there claiming to be anti-aging today but the overwhelming majority have no scientific basis of proof or merit. However, Botox is truly prophylactic. If you have the habit of constantly frowning or raising your eyebrows to make a point, Botox can prevent the wrinkles that result. If the skin around the eyebrows and forehead isn't squeezed like an accordion a few hundred—or thousand—times a day over several years, the skin will not prematurely form an indentation. This benefit holds true for patients of any age. Likewise, if someone has the appearance of two cords running vertically down their neck, especially when speaking loudly, and these muscular cords can be relaxed, then they won't be pulling down and stretching the neck skin over years. This can prevent the premature appearance of a "turkey neck."

I am often asked by patients if they need Botox. There can be only one truthful answer to that question—no. Nobody *needs* Botox. At least no one coming to the office for a cosmetic consultation. But its use can improve the quality of many patients' appearance, and as a result, their lives.

Where Do Wrinkles Come From?

Any given patient's wrinkles probably come from a variety of causes. As we age, the skin becomes less elastic and thinner, so that when it stretches it doesn't snap back like it used to. This causes an excess of skin in certain areas. Also, the fat beneath the skin tends to move downward over the years as it's pulled by gravity. This facial fat also decreases in quantity over the years. Despite what you may think, this is not usually a good thing. Loss of fat under the skin simply makes the amount of excess stretched skin appear even more exaggerated. Even the bones of the face tend to shrink, which can lead to an increase in the appearance of certain lines. Botox has no direct effect on the skin, fat, or bone. It works only on muscles. So how much of a result a patient can expect from a Botox injection depends on how much the visible signs of aging are the result of muscular activity. If a line is half caused by muscular activity and half by hanging, excess skin and fat, a Botox injection will make that line about 50 percent better.

In my practice, there is no upper age limit for Botox injections. The FDA approval for Botox granted in April was limited to the frowning area between the eyebrows in patients under sixty-six years of age. This does not mean that Botox doesn't have a positive effect on seniors. Quite the contrary, I have had excellent results in patients who are in their seventies and eighties. Multiple factors have created the lines for patients in this age group. Stretched thin skin that has been pulled down by gravity over many years also contributes to the depth of the wrinkles. In some cases, if the wrinkles are only 20 percent due to muscular action the patient can expect only about 20 percent improvement with Botox. Generally, the patient is very happy with this 20 percent improvement as long as that is what they were told to expect. Very often, excellent and more dramatic results are achieved by combination therapy. Since an older patient's lines have been there for many years and are very deep, there's an actual dent into the thickness of the skin. Botox combined with a filler material such as collagen or fat will often give great results. In the older patient who has had prior surgery, an even more effective outcome can be obtained. This is because the hanging pulled-down excess skin has been lifted and tightened, making the muscle once again the primary cause of the wrinkles. Too often, physicians and their patients think of Botox in place of surgery or in place of injectable filler materials. Actually, in many patients they work extremely well together.

Public Personas: Actors, Models, and Newscasters

A few years ago, an actress that I dated lamented that she couldn't use Botox. A friend of hers who had used it looked so good. When I asked her why she ruled out Botox, she replied that since she was an actress, obviously she could not afford to have her face paralyzed. She was mistakenly parroting one of the biggest misconceptions about Botox. True, her friend looked her best when she was at rest—when animated, she didn't look exactly natural. But that was the result of poorly done injections rather than anything about Botox itself. And it's not just actors and actresses who feel this way. Recently, film directors Martin Scorsese and Baz Luhrman complained that Botox injections have become so prevalent in Hollywood that it's difficult to find an actress who can fully animate and project her emotions onscreen. And from the look of some actresses and actors, I would agree with them. But the fault lies not with the Botox but with the injector. Botox is simply a tool. It is a tool like collagen is a tool, laser resurfacing is a tool, and a facelift is a tool. Any tool can be used poorly. Everyone has seen bad facelifts, bad nose jobs, bad collagen, and, unfortunately, bad Botox. When collagen, facelifts, and nose jobs look bad, it is usually the result of going too far. The same is true for Botox. I can't tell you how many times I've recommended collagen for the little lines around the mouth and a patient looks at me in horror. They'll tell me that they don't want those huge lips Goldie Hawn had in that movie or Pamela Anderson lips. It takes some time to convince patients that they don't have to look like that. Most people only notice collagen—or Botox—when it has been overdone.

When properly given, Botox injections allow a great deal of control over how much to weaken a muscle. While Botox does paralyze the small part of the muscle whose nerve endings are affected by Botox, a muscle is made up of *thousands* of muscle fibers. So, only a very small minority of the muscle fibers that I inject are paralyzed. You do not have to completely paralyze a muscle to see the beneficial effects of Botox. In fact, I think the best results occur when muscles are only partially weakened.

Even an on-camera performer can have the best of both worlds—and in my practice I see plenty of actors, models, and newscasters. With the muscles slightly weakened and when the face is at rest they have minimal or no lines. But when they animate, their face moves normally. The one downside is that the effect doesn't last as long when Botox is done this way. That is because the nerve fibers that have not been blocked by Botox will reach out and reattach to the sleeping muscle fibers. And there are a lot of live nerve fibers nearby with only a small amount of weakening. So performers often need more frequent Botox injections. In their case, cost and convenience are not nearly as important as appearance. They are certainly willing to have more frequent, lighter injections. But you don't have to be a performer to take advantage of this injection technique. Just ask my office staff. They benefit from cycling Botox injections too. They don't have to worry about the time or expense. I prefer it when my patients have normal motion. And I absolutely want everyone in my office looking natural. I don't want my patients to think that a pack of zombies is responsible for their care or that they'll end up looking as if they walked off the set of *The Stepford Wives*. The trickle-down effect may not be evident today in the field of economics but it is alive and well in the fields of plastic surgery and dermatology. Just as some of the worst hair plugs I have ever seen are on display on the scalps of hair transplant surgeons, some of the strangest expressions—or lack of them—belong to the faces of Botox injectors. Cycling is good for anyone whose primary concern is appearance and not the time, pain, or expense of injections.

Actors will often time their Botox injections around a project. Frequently, they will keep the muscles very weakened for a period of time before shooting. This gives the skin a chance to heal itself without being puckered a few thousand times a day. The skin is a living, dynamic organ. When the repetitive trauma of being scrunched over and over is removed, it can actually repair itself. The period when the muscles are starting to regain strength is the perfect time to be caught on film. Lines at rest are greatly diminished due to the muscles' slightly weakened state and also due to the vacation from crackling that the skin has just enjoyed. Yet when animated, a natural expression and range of emotion is the result.

The Post-Lift Patient

When we were talking about the slightly older patient earlier in the chapter, I discussed how sometimes in our later years Botox can have a decreasing efficacy. This is due most commonly to excess skin and sagging fat. The effect of Botox can have several peaks over a lifetime. The first peak occurs in the younger patient whose lines are formed almost entirely by muscular action. This effect diminishes as the skin begins to stretch. Secondary peaks occur in the older patient who has already had a face and neck lift as well as possibly a browlift and eyelid surgery. These surgical procedures tighten and remove excess skin while lifting the descended fat and muscles beneath the skin. Since in these patients their lines are visible again primarily due to muscular action, Botox has a greater effect. So while Botox has been used across the board in my practice for patients in their twenties through their mid-eighties, there are two peaks when its effects are maximized: patients in their thirties and forties without a great deal of sagging skin and fat and patients at any age who have had the excess skin and fat lifted and smoothed. This is especially true for the neck. As I said before, the younger patient will often have two cords running down the neck when speaking strongly. Botox can eliminate these lines in these patients. However, as that patient ages, especially if that patient has not been injecting these cords and these cords have stretched the skin of the neck, Botox will have only a minimal effect. Botox will not elevate or tighten this sagging skin. But after the skin and the muscles of the neck have been tightened, these cords will disappear. No surgical procedure can stop the aging process or the effect of gravity on the neck. After several years these cords can start to return. When this happens, Botox again becomes an excellent treatment for these cords since they are made of muscle and the skin is still relatively taut from the prior surgery. This is also very true for the fan-shaped areas on the outer edge of the eyes commonly called crow's feet. For the younger patient, injection of the crow's feet often yields dramatic improvement and even elimination of these lines. But as that patient ages some excess skin of the upper and lower eyelids can coalesce in this area. This excess skin limits the effectiveness of Botox. But after an eyelid tuck, this excess skin is reduced and Botox again becomes an excellent treatment for this area.

It's not only that Botox works better in the older patient who has been lifted, but also that it can extend the life of that lift. Think about it. Once the last stitch has been put in on the operating table, the clock starts ticking again. Sure, if your surgeon was good maybe you've turned the clock back a few years. Well, what's wrong with making it run more slowly? The muscles that support your chin and neck have just been tightened. Do you really want them to start pulling down again immediately? The skin around your eyes after a combination of surgery and laser resurfacing is beautifully smooth. Do you really want it to be severely crinkled tomorrow? Once again Botox and surgery are not mutually exclusive. While some patients can delay surgery for a few years due to its effects, just because you've finally had the surgery is no reason to abandon your Botox. Surgery, by reducing excess skin and tightening lax muscle, can help your Botox work better and your Botox just may keep the results of your surgery looking fresh for a few extra years.

Notox

Botox is, sadly, not for everyone. Patients with neuromuscular disorders such as myasthenia gravis, Lambert-Eaton syndrome, or ALS (also known as Lou Gehrig disease) should not be injected. Certain antibiotics also preclude its use. I do not inject women who are pregnant, trying to become pregnant, or nursing. If you are unsure, you should discuss these issues carefully with your physician.

3

THE BOTOX RX

Stop Scowling

The first area of the face I ever injected with Botox was that between the eyebrows. My first patient was considering a two-hour operation that would include an incision from ear to ear across the top of her head, folding her forehead down over her face (not unlike being scalped), surgically removing the frowning muscles from beneath the eyebrows, then putting her back together with a row of metal staples across the top of her head. So it was natural that I chose these frowning muscles to be the first that I would inject with Botox. That is because these muscles were routinely removed and thrown away during a very popular operation of the early 1990s. People who'd had these muscles removed did very well without them so I figured that having these muscles at least partially paralyzed would look good too. As expected, these early patients were unable to frown after their Botox injections. The improvement in their appearance while frowning (or attempting to frown) was dramatic.

What was not so expected was the tremendous improvement in their appearance at rest. Patients who had some fine to moderate frown lines present even while not frowning had these resting frown lines eliminated. There are two good reasons why this happens. One, even when at rest— when you are not angry, not emotional, not squinting or trying to frown— the frowning muscles have a certain resting tone. That is, they are always pulling and contracting a tiny bit, even when you're asleep. Botox produces smoothing of the skin even at rest. I think that as we age, this resting tone of the muscles increases relative to the skin's ability to resist it. That, coupled with the downward pull of gravity on the tissues of the eyebrows, leads to an increase in the frown lines. That's why even seniors with very pronounced frown lines can get such a good result from Botox injections in this area. Two, by preventing the frowning muscles from crumpling the skin between the brows several thousand times a day, Botox allows the skin to heal itself. If the skin has been severely damaged by the sun or cigarette-smoking, Botox at least prevents the muscles from making the skin even worse. What many people and even their doctors fail to realize is that the skin is a living, dynamic organ. It is, in fact, the largest organ of the body. This dynamic tissue has a tremendous ability to heal itself, and it helps to explain the increased improvement seen when Botox is used consistently over many years.

Often when frown lines are very deep and have been present for many years, Botox cannot eliminate them at first. The wrinkle is just too deep and too established to simply disappear. But Botox can at least make that wrinkle less visible. After doing this for so many years, I can guess fairly accurately if a line will go way or just be improved. As long as patients know ahead of time that the line may be only reduced and not erased, they are very happy with the improvement they get. Occasionally, I will recommend that the patient have another treatment in addition to Botox. This is usually an in-office injection of a filler material such as collagen.

Filler materials have a totally different mechanism of action than Botox does. The filler material is injected into the skin, not the muscle. It physically takes up space and pumps up the skin. This makes for an excellent secondary procedure in the patient with heavy, established wrinkles. Botox relaxes the muscle that was the primary cause for the line in the first place. But since the line is so deep, it will not be erased. Then, by putting a filler material into the skin this deep wrinkle can be plumped up and eliminated. Very often, when I can tell that the wrinkle is much too deep to be removed by Botox, I will recommend and inject both the Botox and the collagen at the same treatment session. Sometimes, patients want to wait and see how much better just the Botox alone will make them. So I will inject them with Botox and they can decide for themselves after about a week if the Botox made the wrinkle less noticeable enough to make them happy. If not, the patient will come back for a quick visit, at which time I'll put a little collagen beneath the wrinkle, smoothing it out. The patient in Figs. 97 and 98 had frown lines that were almost completely eliminated by Botox. On a different office visit, she had a filler material injected beneath the fine remaining wrinkles to eliminate them.

Before Botox came along, there were already many treatments for frown lines. Collagen injections, fat injections, dermabrasion, chemical peels, and brow-lift surgery were common treatments for the brow area. These are still good treatments for the brow area, and laser resurfacing has been added to our tool kit. But if I had to choose only one treatment for frown lines, it would certainly be Botox. And when I realize that patients will need a combination of treatments to achieve the result they're looking for, Botox is still the first line of defense. Theoretically, it makes sense: the root cause of frown lines begins and ends with the muscle wrinkling the skin. And practically, it will give the best result of any single treatment other than surgery. I think it's a disservice to the patient if surgery is recommended first when the problem could possibly be corrected or at least improved with Botox. I know what you're thinking. That everyone knows about Botox and who in their right mind would initially request surgery to improve their frown lines when Botox is so readily available. But you have to remember that I've been injecting Botox since 1991 and it hasn't always been so popular. Many surgeons continued to recommend brow surgery as a primary treatment even though they knew that Botox could give the patient an excellent result. The problem was, many patients had not yet heard of Botox and didn't request it prior to their surgery. I certainly think it's appropriate to use brow surgery as a first-line treatment if Botox and its potential benefits are at least discussed with the patient beforehand. Some patients prefer the surgery so that they don't have to go to the doctor every few months for several tiny injections. Also, for the *severely* wrinkled brow, surgery gives a better result than Botox. But surgery has its downside as well. Obviously it's more invasive than Botox and you have to carve on average two weeks out of your life for recovery. There are four basic variations of brow surgery. The first, a coronal browlift, involves a long incision across the top of the head. A coronal browlift usually completely removes the frowning muscles and also elevates the brows with a fair amount of precision. Another procedure, called an endoscopic browlift, uses five smaller incisions of about a half inch each across the top of the head. Using a tiny camera mounted to a lens via a long narrow tube, long curved instruments, and a video screen, the surgeon can delicately pluck out the frowning muscles bit by bit while watching his video screen. During the surgery with the surgeon staring at the screen, not the patient, it actually looks as though the surgeon is playing a video game. Third, the frowning muscles can also be removed through an incision in the upper eyelid, called "transpalpebral corrugator resection." This approach is usually taken if the patient is having upper eyelid surgery because the muscles can be removed through the same incision. However, this surgery doesn't directly elevate the brows. The newer, fourth approach to these muscles, which I call "direct corrugator excision" is more direct. I make a small incision directly through the eyebrow straight down to these muscles, which are then partially removed. Using these last two direct approaches, the brows are not directly elevated and all of the muscle cannot be removed easily. And that is how they are explained to the patient. Where I think some patients have been sold a bill of goods, however, is with the endoscopic browlift. When this operation first became very popular in the early and mid-'90s, I saw many presentations by excellent surgeons about it at medical meetings.

As with any new procedure, the complications were extensively discussed. But what I felt was not discussed was the fact that it was extremely difficult and a little dangerous to try to remove *all* of the frowning muscles by this approach. In fact, I do not tell my patients who are about to undergo this surgery that they won't be able to frown or wrinkle their brows again. I simply make those muscles a bit weaker by removing just a bit of them. Actually, a lot of patients like that. They want to have some motion and some ability to frown and look angry; they just want their lines to look better.

Unfortunately, many surgeons are apparently not so forthcoming with their patients. Either that, or they honestly overestimate their ability to remove these muscles through an endoscopic browlift. I have many disappointed patients in my practice who had an endoscopic browlift elsewhere, when they were told that they would never need to have another Botox injection to this area or the forehead again. That is rarely the case. There's just about always some muscle left and some movement—sometimes so little muscle that Botox is not needed again. But in many cases Botox is needed to maximize the cosmetic appearance of the brow. It all depends on how much muscle is left and how it is left. If only a very small amount is left and the contour of the skin of the brow looks good, all is well. But if only a little muscle is left and an indentation exists, this dent will be greatly magnified by even a small amount of muscle. There is even more of a problem when there are little pieces of the muscle left irregularly along the brow. This can lead to a strange pattern of dents and irregular motion across the brow. The other problem with this is that injecting Botox into these patients is frequently much more painful than in a patient who has not had brow surgery. The reason is the scar tissue. Scar tissue is tough, dense, and very inelastic. When Botox is injected into a muscle, it makes that muscle swell up, increasing its volume temporarily. That can be fairly painful when a muscle is trapped by scar tissue that just won't stretch.

Another good use for Botox in the forehead is in the patient who has had a browlift gone awry. I don't mean with just a little extra muscle left behind as described above. That is not what I'd consider a complication, just a limitation of the surgery. One problem in particular was very common around 1995 when this procedure was relatively new and gaining in popularity. I was referred many patients who had the double whammy of still retaining much of their frowning musculature as well as having dents created between the eyes. This was a relatively new technique and a new way of operating for many surgeons. And in their attempt to remove all the musculature, sometimes they would be a little aggressive and actually remove part of the undersurface of the skin or the fat beneath it. This would create a dent and when coupled with a still strong muscle, a really deep, deep frown line. Not many plastic surgeons were doing Botox yet in those years, so a lot of these patients were referred to me. Their treatment was twofold: Botox injections to relax the still-present muscle and fat injections to refill the volume lost. The results of this combination therapy were excellent. Without Botox, many of these patients would have been subjected to additional surgery, which would have been made much more difficult due to the scar tissue from the first operation. Just think, not only would the surgeon have to deal with a lot of dense scar tissue but the muscle that he was looking for would have been smaller and irregularly placed. Add to this the fact that some fat or deep skin might have already been removed and you have a setup for not just a residual dent but a real problem.

The patient in Figs. 101 and 102 had exactly this problem. She had an endoscopic browlift that left behind a fair amount of muscle pulling her brows together. Just at the inside edge of each brow she was left with a dent. In the dented area there was no muscle, making the appearance of the dent more obvious. She also did not get much of a browlift. Her brows were in the same low, flat position that they started in. She was a good patient for both Botox and fat injection. With Botox preventing the frown muscles from working and the fat filling up the dents left by overzealous removal of tissue, this patient had a much smoother brow.

It was in these endoscopic browlift patients that I realized another tremendous benefit of Botox. Through the early '90s, I had thought that when they were used together Botox increased the longevity of a filler material such as collagen. But that is something that is very difficult to quantify or prove. How do you know how much collagen is still left deep down in the skin? I also thought that Botox added tremendously to the longevity of fat injections. But it was in these specific patients that I saw the true answer. I have never had to repeat, redo, or give a booster injection of fat to the frown lines in any patient who has been conscientious in keeping up with the Botox and preventing full muscular return. I have given additional fat injections to these patients, but never to the area between the eyes if it has been kept relatively immobile with Botox. Without the constant folding, wrinkling, and crushing motion on the filler materials created by the musculature, those filler materials last a great deal longer.

The patient in Figs. 103 and 104 had the same problem but to a more severe extent. Her muscle removal was much more irregular with intermittent areas of full strength and no motion at all. She also had two much larger, irregularly shaped dents where all of her muscle and possibly some fat and deep skin were removed. This was more of a challenge. Her motion and contour defects were very irregular. Even finding the small pieces of muscle was tricky. I try to avoid injecting the entire area in these patients, as the injections are much more painful than in the patient who has not had surgery. Filling these irregular dents with fat can also be a challenge, but this patient had an excellent result. She is frowning in both pictures. The patient in Figs. 101 and 102 recently had repeat fat injections, but not to her brow area. Fat was injected into her smile lines, but despite the fact that her brow fat injections were six years old, they did not need any booster fat.

Watching patients' frown lines over many years led me to another discovery about the beneficial effects of Botox. Even the patient with established frown lines whose lines are improved but not eliminated with Botox receives an extra benefit from the Botox. Say this patient did not want a simultaneous treatment such as injection of collagen. Sure, the lines were still there, but they were minimized and so the patient didn't want any additional treatment other than regular Botox injections. I have had many of these patients in my practice for several years. About 1994,

I realized something truly remarkable. Very slowly over several years, if patients prevent the muscles from coming back full strength, the original deep line which was minimized to a moderate or fine line by Botox actually gets *better* over the years. That's a testament to the tremendous healing ability of skin, which can actually remodel itself over many years and look better and better with time. It's quite remarkable to look at frown lines or the forehead area or crow's feet area of a patient and note that the area without surgery, just with Botox injections, actually looks better ten years later than it did at the start of Botox treatment. And I don't mean just from the weakening affect of Botox on the muscles. That would be an unfair comparison. When I say that an area looks better after ten years I don't mean the area initially uninjected compared to the area ten years older after it's been injected. That would be easy. The weakening affect of Botox on the muscles alone would make the skin look better. What I'm talking about is comparing the brow or forehead of someone with the full Botox effect on board ten years ago to the same area again with full Botox on board ten years later. Or comparing a person immediately before a Botox injection to the same person before injection many years later. Most of these patients have had truly remarkable age-defying results by keeping up with their injections. This effect is demonstrated in Figs. 83–88. This patient is five years older in her photos on the right. In both sets of photos she has not had a recent injection. The photos on the left show her prior to her first injection, and the photos on the right show her one year after her last injection.

Of all the areas that I have injected, the frown lines are the only ones that I feel comfortable paralyzing. You hear that word a lot in association with Botox. In fact, only a very small percentage of the muscles that I inject are truly paralyzed. I think that most muscles need only to be somewhat weakened or relaxed to give the best results possible. Most patients are not unhappy with the inability to frown or look angry. Most of them think that this is an additional benefit. I have had countless patients tell me that they get along with people better at work and people seem to treat them better after their Botox injections. That's because some people have a tendency to frown or scowl all the time, not only when they are angry or cross. Even patients without that tendency some-times develop that look simply because they have fairly strong muscles in the frowning area. People with muscles that powerful have a stronger resting tone in the muscles so they nearly always appear to be scowling. These patients have told me that Botox was an almost life-changing event for them. People in sales frequently report that Botox for them is not a luxury but a requirement for their job. Suppose you needed to buy a product and there were two on the market nearly identical in quality and price. One company had a salesman who was relaxed and sincere. The other company had a salesman who constantly looked as though he were about to explode or at least scream at you if you didn't choose his product. Which company's product would you choose?

Another unique aspect of injecting Botox into the frown muscles is, unfortunately, the pain. Of all the different areas that I have injected, most patients would vote for this area as the most painful. There are several reasons for this. For Botox to work its best, it must be directly injected into the muscle. The muscles in this area are deep, lying right on top of the bone. It requires a pretty deep injection. Another reason for the sensitivity is the abundance of sensory nerves in this area. You may recall the two distinct types of nerves in the human body from chapter 1. The sensory nerves relay impulses from the skin toward the brain, bringing it information from the skin. These are the nerves re-sponsible for our sense of touch and feeling and pain. These nerves are not affected by Botox. But when a great many of these nerves converge in one area it becomes very sensitive. There are two bundles of such nerves on each side of the brow going in through a small hole in the bone toward the brain. Unfortunately, these nerves course directly through the body of one of the muscles that is injected to reduce frown lines. To say that this is a sensitive area would be an understatement. Occasionally patients will feel what they describe as an electric shock going up the forehead during injection into this area. This happens when the needle entering the muscle actually touches one of the nerve fibers.

You may have read something about Botox and migraine headaches. There are several studies in the literature that show partial improvement in migraine headache sufferers after Botox injections. The mechanism for this is not completely understood. However, most experts agree that migraine headaches can be triggered by irritating some of these four nerve bundles that course through the frowning muscles. It is thought that when these nerves are disturbed they release a substance that can trigger a migraine headache. So it makes sense that if the muscles through which these nerves course are paralyzed then there is less of a chance that muscular action could irritate these nerves and trigger a headache. Again, anatomy is the key to understanding. The nerve as it comes through the small opening in the bone is fixed. There is no give in the bone. It is solid. But as soon as the nerve peeks out from the bone, it is in the middle of a very active muscle that pulls sharply on the nerve side to side, stretching (nerves are not very elastic) the nerve, irritating it. My patients who are true migraine headache sufferers usually do derive some benefit from Botox. Most patients say that since they've been having the injections their migraine headaches certainly appear to occur less often. I've never had a patient whose migraine headaches were cured or never recurred due to Botox injections. These patients also observe that when they do get a migraine headache it appears to be less severe than the headaches they used to get before they started Botox injections. If for cosmetic reasons I'm injecting a patient who has severe migraines, I will often inject the muscles in the temple as well, since these muscles are also thought to trigger migraines. (One word of caution here. I am talking about true migraine headaches. Due to blanket advertising of many headache remedies, many people are under the impression that any really severe headache is a migraine headache. That is not so. They are different conditions with different causes.)

But just as Botox injections can reduce the frequency and severity of migraine headaches, they can also cause regular headaches. In fact, in Allergan's FDA study, headache was the most frequently reported side effect after Botox injections. In the company study the quoted headache rate was 15 percent. I feel that the post-injection headache is caused by two factors that can be very nearly eliminated. I've never done a scientific study of all my patients, but I do see them frequently and I can assure you that their headache rate after injection is very small, probably close to 1 or 2 percent. One way that headaches can be generated in the injection process is by tension and by patients' breathing patterns. I try to get my patients to relax before their injections. I do this by laying them back and not shining a bright light into their eyes. I also talk them through the procedure, letting them know what I'm going to do without sneaking up on them. Something else that I feel is very important is a patient's breathing pattern during injection. Some patients tend to hold their breath and really bear down when they experience any pain. I think breath-holding and bearing down trigger a lot of the post-injection headaches. I try to get my patients to close their eyes, relax, and breathe slowly and deeply through the mouth during their injections. It's almost like yoga breathing. Very often, I have to remind my patients to breathe during the injections as some people tend to hold their breath. Another possible mechanism for the creation of headaches is when the injection is not done very well by the injector. I said previously that the frowning muscles to be injected are deep, lying right on top of the bone. That's not exactly true. The bone has a thin, tough covering that is wrapped around it. This covering is extremely sensitive. Any irritation of this covering can cause a great deal of pain and, I believe, headache. Unfortunately, the muscles are right on top of this covering. I think very frequently an injector will jab the needle into this covering, which causes a great deal of pain and can trigger headaches. I've even heard a Botox "expert" telling other doctors that the way to inject Botox accurately is to insert the needle until it hits this covering, then back up a little bit to be sure that the needle tip is in the muscle. While that might make it easier to find the muscle, I don't think that it's a good technique. Certainly, I have hit my share of the bone's wrapping with a needle. But after thousands of patients, I can fairly easily put that needle right down to but not quite touching the covering. This spares my patients the additional pain caused by pinching this membrane.

What proof do I have that these two factors cause the headaches and not the Botox itself? For one thing, there was a control group in the study. That is, certain patients were injected but there was no Botox in the solution. But neither the patients nor the injectors knew who was getting Botox and who was not. This assured that the patients would be injected in the same manner. The patients who were injected but without Botox also had a headache rate of 15 percent.

Not all Botox injections for frown lines are exactly the same. There are actually eleven different muscle fiber groups that can cause frown lines. How much you weaken or paralyze these eleven segments determines what kind of result you will get. When some people frown, their eyebrows come together and actually turn up toward their forehead as opposed to down. In these patients I will weaken only the segments pulling the brows together and let the other segments naturally raise the brows a bit. I think this gives most patients a better result. Occasionally, a male patient will request that I stop his brows from turning up toward the center of his forehead, saying that it gives him an almost pleading appearance. One of the benefits of beginning to give Botox injections while I was still doing my fellowship at the Manhattan Eye, Ear and Throat Hospital was the incredible amount of surgical experience I gained there. Operating all day with the nation's preeminent plastic surgeons allowed me to look at the musculature of many patients each day. I began to develop a true appreciation for the tremendous variation in anatomy from patient to patient, especially regarding the facial musculature. People whose faces typically moved in certain ways had different underlying muscle patterns. Not all frowning muscles are the same and so they should not be injected the same way. Most men have much longer frowning muscles that attach to the skin toward the middle or outside part of the eyebrow. Most women have shorter muscles that attach to the inner third of the eyebrow. But not always. Some women have frowning musculature that goes nearly to the outer end of their eyebrow whereas some men have a much shorter muscle. By having the patient produce several expressions in a row, based on my surgical experience, I can make a pretty good guess as to where these muscles are. That is the key to performing good Botox injections. The injector must be able to visualize the muscles under the skin. And not just where the muscles are. The injector should also be able to determine which muscles or even parts of muscles are the stronger or more dominant parts and which parts are also present anatomically but do little to determine the patient's pattern of motion.

Despite this fact, many experts and teachers of Botox technique trot out the same tired diagram of a patient's eyebrows with X's or spots for the sites to be injected. Some even list the dose to be injected into each predetermined site. This would work really well if everyone's muscles were in exactly the same place, with exactly the same strength, and everyone made exactly the same types of expression. Obviously we do not. Everyone's patterns are unique and so each patient's injection pattern and dose should also be unique.

For instance, some patients have frowning muscles that pull down the portions of the eyebrows closer to the nose more than other patients. If these muscles are completely paralyzed, those patients will experience an upraising of the inner portion of their eyebrows. Most people want to raise the middle portion of their eyebrows, but not everyone—especially men. Some patients' muscles barely pull the eyebrows down at all, but instead tend to pull them together. This should be recognized beforehand so that patients aren't erroneously told that they will receive a mild lifting of the brows after their injections.

Signing Off

Clearly, it is of paramount importance to recognize the frowning patterns of individual patients. Some patients scrunch up the bridge of their nose so much when frowning that it almost looks as though they're smelling something unpleasant. I've heard several Botox experts talk about the "Botox sign." This, they say, is the telltale sign that someone has had Botox. It occurs when all the frowning muscles have been paralyzed except for the small muscles on each side of the upper bridge of the nose. When certain people frown these muscles are very active, though for most people they are not. When these patients' frowning muscles can no longer move, these patients actually recruit these muscles to try to frown, thereby giving rise to the "Botox sign," or excessive wrinkling across the top of the nose. My patients don't get the "Botox sign." That's because since 1992, most patients who appear prone to wrinkle in this area get a few extra drops of Botox on each side of the nose. But I do not inject everybody this way. Some patients want a very dramatic arch in their brows, so I deliberately let this muscle along the sides of the nose pull down on the inner part of the brow so the outer raising of the brow looks even more dramatic. Also, why pinch everyone an extra few times when most people will not get the sign? So I'm not going to tell you that I have *never* given one of my patients the "Botox sign." But I'd say on average it happens only about once a year. And patients who are predisposed to developing the sign are warned about it and encouraged to return to the office if they see it. When the patient comes back into the office, I can fix it in about thirty seconds.

The patient in Figs. 1 through 4 had this pattern of injection. A quick glance at her before photos both at rest and especially while frowning show heavy horizontal wrinkles at the bridge of her nose. If her Botox had been injected in the "standard" pattern often drawn in articles, these lines would not have been improved and she definitely would have had the "Botox sign." Instead, the entire central third of her face looks noticeably smoother. Her fine wrinkles are gone.

Reducing Worry (Lines)

Another excellent target for Botox injection is the muscle that causes the horizontal (or worry) lines across the forehead. According to anatomy textbooks, there are two paired muscles, one on each side of the forehead, that pull up on the eyebrows, raising them. This motion creates horizontal worry lines. After seeing the forehead muscles of thousands of patients, I can tell you that two separate muscles are rarely seen. While I was a fellow at Manhattan Eye, Ear and Throat, the coronal forehead lift was still an extremely popular operation. Before going into the operating room I would routinely mark the worry lines as well as the frown lines with a felt marker on the skin of each patient. Once they were asleep, the muscles beneath these areas would be marked with a needle covered with a small amount of blue liquid, which would dissolve and be gone after a few hours. The blue liquid was a temporary tattoo to guide us to the most active portions of the muscles. Rarely would a patient actually have the classic pattern of two muscles, one on each side of the forehead. Usually, the muscle appeared to be one large horizontally-oriented rectangle. Sure, the muscle tended to be a little thinner toward the outside and right down the middle, but not always. Sometimes the strongest portion of the muscle was right in the middle. Looking at these muscles all day and then injecting Botox late in the afternoon really helped me to appreciate the differences not just in anatomy but also in how these muscles move even when they appear anatomically very similar.

So, since the rectangular forehead muscle pulls up on the eyebrows and wrinkles the skin, weakening that muscle decreases its upward pull on the eyebrows and decreases your horizontal wrinkles. Unfortunately, with the rapid increase in popularity of Botox over the last few years, I think this area tends to be injected more and more poorly. I've seen some patients whose forehead muscle has been completely paralyzed. When this occurs, you lose not only your expression but your natural appearance. When people speak, they tend to move their eyebrows. If you are having a conversation, laughing, or feeling surprised and your eyebrows don't move it all, you tend to look like a statue. Or someone who has recently had a stroke. Neither is a good alternative.

I feel very strongly that the forehead muscle should be only partially weakened. Besides leaving you with a natural appearance, having some of the muscle working gives you an additional benefit. This, after all, is the muscle that raises your eyebrows. If it is severely weakened or paralyzed it will no longer be able to hold your eyebrows up. And I don't just mean when you intentionally raise your eyebrows. Remember that all of these facial muscles have a certain resting tone. Even when you're relaxed, the muscle is always pulling up a little bit. So if you eliminate that resting tone, not only will you be unable to express surprise or feign interest when your lunch date is telling you another endless story about work, but even when resting, your eyebrows will flatten out and sit lower on your forehead. Sometimes much lower on the forehead, possibly even so low that your eyebrows will actually hold your eyelids down, making you feel very tired at the end of the day. Most women's eyebrows are at or slightly above the bony ridge of the eye socket, which you can easily feel above your eye. Most men's eyebrows are at or just below this ridge. Dropping a woman's brow below this ridge or a man's brow even lower can create an extremely unappealing appearance. You may not want to look like Alfred E. Neuman but you don't want to look like the one person at work who can't keep their eyes open either.

Different sections of the forehead muscle dominate in different people. Usually, the heaviest worry lines are across the middle section of the forehead. But not always. Sometimes the outer portion of the muscle is strongest, leaving the heavier wrinkles above the outer eyebrows. Every patient is different, and having a standardized pattern of forehead injection is ridiculous. The injections must be tailored to each individual patient depending on how strong the muscle is and where the stronger versus weaker sections are. If the muscle's strength is fairly evenly spread out, I prefer to weaken the central portion more than the outer portion in most people. When people speak to each other, they tend to focus on the central areas of the face, so for most people, I prefer to smooth the center of the forehead, leaving a few shallower lines closer to the temples.

Injecting this area also carries with it the risk of increasing the appearance of asymmetry. No one's face is completely symmetrical and the same is true for worry lines. The first time I treat a patient, I nearly always inject the forehead evenly on each side. Despite that fact, about 5 percent of patients will be able to raise one eyebrow much more strongly than the other after that injection. This is what I call the "Groucho" effect. The reason is the muscle in their forehead has always been stronger on one side than the other. But since even the weaker side was fairly strong, the disparity was never readily apparent. But with the muscle weakened, the difference in strength is magnified and one side raises and wrinkles more than the other. Luckily, this condition is very simple to fix. Just another drop of Botox in the stronger side can even you back out. After years of experience, I now frequently inject even first-time patients asymmetrically. Although their foreheads may seem symmetrical to them, I can sometimes detect a difference in strength between the two sides that would potentially be magnified after the injection. Giving the strong side a little extra Botox at the first injection saves the patient from having to come back into the office for a touch-up injection. I call this differential weakening. The clearest example of this asymmetry is when a person (other than Groucho) can strongly raise just one eyebrow at a time. Someone who can do that can almost always only do it with just one eyebrow and not both. That side is much stronger even if the worry lines appear to be the same on each side. The trick is in finding patients who have a less noticeable degree of asymmetry beforehand. If you have a tendency toward asymmetry, that will reveal itself after your first completely symmetrical injection. If you go back to let your physician examine you and fix the problem, it shouldn't happen again. That's one advantage of sticking with one injector and not jumping from doctor to doctor for your injections. I feel that I do a slightly better job on patients I have been injecting for many years each year that goes by.

The forehead area was the second area that I ever injected in a person. Very often, during the coronal browlift operation, the large muscle in the forehead is partially weakened. Usually this is done by excising small parts of the muscle. To avoid irregular motion, the muscle is not completely removed in one section and allowed to stay at full strength in another. Instead, I shave off large areas of muscle but in very thin slices at a time. That way you have a normal motion pattern but with an overall weakness (at least all over where the shaving was done). Milder weakening is done through lightly breaking up the muscle fibers by dividing them in a checkerboard pattern. Alternatively, the muscle is just touched in a few spots with the machine we use to cauterize blood vessels, which results in an even smaller amount of weakening. The key is to follow the little temporary tattoos made before the start of the operation. They guide me to where I want the muscle weakened. That, combined with differential weakening, gives me control over the forehead. So really, I was just duplicating, on a temporary basis with an injection, what I had been doing night and day in the operating room.

Differential weakening is the key to consistently good results in a wide variety of different patients. Most commonly I weaken the center of the forehead a bit more than the other areas. But not always. Sometimes the weakening is evenly distributed, sometimes more along the outside, sometimes more across the upper or lower forehead, sometimes in an irregular pattern depending on the wrinkle pattern, shape of the face, size of the forehead, or position of the eyebrows.

The woman in Figs. 9 through 14 is in her mid-fifties. When frowning, she had very heavy lines both between her eyes and at the top of her nose that were removed with Botox. Looking at her forehead in Fig. 11, you can see that she has the most common type of wrinkle pattern. Her lines are heaviest down the middle of the forehead and fade over the outer third of the brows. They are also different vertically. Right down the middle, she has no lines over the lower third of her forehead (this also allows us to see just how heavy her left frown line is when her frown muscles are resting and the skin is even being stretched upward). On top of her brows, the lines go right down to the brow. She has a high forehead and flat brows.

Her upper middle forehead was heavily weakened, above the brows was lightly weakened, and outside the brows minimally weakened. But this was not done evenly on both sides. When you see her face at rest in Fig. 13, you can see that her left brow sits a little lower and flatter than her right. So, on the left side of her forehead, I left her a little stronger, especially over the middle portion of her brow. When I raised her brows after injection, you can see in Fig. 12 that her left brow peaks closer to its center than the right, which peaks more toward the outside of the brow. I wanted to get her left brow up and more arched.

The before-and-after photos at rest in Figs. 13 and 14 tell the end of the story. Despite being deeply ingrained, her frown lines were nearly gone. If she wanted further improvement, collagen would have been my first choice to fill in the slight depression that remains. Her left brow has more muscle pulling up on it so it is higher and more arched over its center and much more symmetric than before. If she had been injected using a "standard" pattern, her brow asymmetry would be worse and her brows would be flatter and lower. This patient also had a slightly droopy left eyelid before injection, which almost certainly would have given her a completely droopy eyelid after injection if her injections were not highly individualized. Instead, her droopy lid is actually *less* noticeable than before.

Sometimes the reason that a forehead is severely wrinkled lies not in the forehead itself but in the area a little lower on the face. Some patients have a large amount of heavy skin in the upper eyelid. This weight sits across the top of their eyelids. To say that the eyelids do not appreciate this kind of treatment is an understatement. The eyelid-raising muscle and other structures in the eyelids are extremely delicate. To relieve their burden they send a signal to the forehead muscles to lift the heavy skin off them. This feels great. The muscle is relieved. For about a minute. Then that heavy skin starts to slide back down on top of the lid and the cycle repeats itself. All that lifting by the forehead sure beats up your skin in a hurry. Usually, removing that heavy skin with surgery not only makes your eyes look a lot better, but it also keeps your forehead from scrunching itself up so it looks a lot better too. Sometimes, the cycle of sensing the weight of the skin followed by lifting is so deeply ingrained that it continues even though the weight is gone. Very often, Botox can break this now unecessary habit after one or two injections.

Most patients will say that the forehead is the second most tender area to have injected. While the sensory nerves in the forehead aren't quite as dense as they are in the frowning area, there are still several nerve bundles that course through the forehead. In addition, the muscles in the forehead are fairly deep as well.

Sometimes I get a little resistance from patients who only want their forehead to be injected. In 1991, I had injected a few patients only in their forehead because they didn't really have any other creases that bothered them. But these patients did not look very good after their injections. Sure, their horizontal wrinkles were much better, but there was something unappealing about their appearance.

One of the potential problems that I envisioned before beginning to inject Botox was a condition called eyelid ptosis. This was a problem that many patients had encountered if they had Botox injected very close to their eye for muscle spasms. The muscle that raises your eyelids and opens your eyes is not very large or strong. If a little Botox were to seep in there, it could cause your upper eyelid to droop. Before injecting anyone, I developed several strategies to prevent this unwanted occurrence. I had injected a young woman in her thirties about five days before I got the phone call. "I'm having trouble keeping my eyes open," she said. I figured that I had somehow gotten some Botox into her eyelid-raising muscle. When I examined her, her eyelid muscles seemed to work fine and her eyelids were in good position, not drooping. But she looked odd and tired nonetheless. That's because her brows had become flattened and lowered, even though I left part of the muscle in the forehead working. The problem was due to an imbalance of the muscles. In the last section, I discussed how the frowning muscles can strongly pull down the ends of the eyebrows closest to the nose. If these muscles are left at full strength and their opposing muscle in the forehead trying to raise the brows is weakened, an imbalance results. The muscles pulling down on the brow begin to dominate and the brow is lowered. Since 1992, even if patients want only their forehead to be injected, I insist on injecting their frowning muscles, which is not a routine practice. Most injectors working today will inject only the forehead if the patient requests it. I would say that is unfortunate. I can't tell you how many patients I've had in my office for the first time tell me Botox doesn't work for them in their forehead. When I ask why, they usually tell me that they'd had it done and their eyebrows became too low and flattened and their physician told them they were not good candidates for the procedure. Almost every time I've been told this story, when I asked the patients if they had their eyebrows or bridge of the nose injected at the same time, they looked at me quizzically and said no. Sometimes, I'll have a new patient who doesn't want the frowning areas injected, just the forehead. These patients are sometimes a lot harder to convince. That was one of the reasons that I changed my fee schedule for Botox injections. Since the frown area and forehead are the most common areas injected, my basic Botox injection includes those two areas. I don't want a patient to not want the frowning area injected with Botox solely because of money. So my lowest fee always includes a minimum of two areas, which has made it easier for me to do the right thing for a few had-to-convince patients.

The patient in Figs. 35 and 36 wanted her outer eyebrows to come up a bit and did not like her worry lines, which she first noticed four years before. She had a very youthful appearance and she thought these lines made her look nervous or unsure of herself. Only the middle of the forehead was weakened, which impelled her outer forehead to pull up harder. The permanent look of concern that she had is gone.

The next patient, in Figs. 37 and 38, did not have any weakening of her middle forehead. That, coupled with paralyzing her frown muscles, allowed her inner brows to spring up.

Even though the patient in Figs. 39 through 42 had just turned thirty, she had fairly strong wrinkle lines across her forehead. These lines did not make her face appear nervous or worried, just a bit tired. Her forehead was weakened almost uniformly across, as her lines are nearly uniformly deep across her forehead. I also wanted to emphasize her bright blue eyes and so I gave her a little less Botox directly over the middle of each eyebrow.

Another interesting and pleasant byproduct of Botox injections in this area has to do with scars. As opposed to what many patients think, scars are living, dynamic stretches of tissue upon normal skin. Scars change over time. Typically, they tend to get a little shorter as they slowly contract over many years. One thing that can make a scar heal poorly is tension on the skin. Whenever the skin is cut, scar tissue is the only way that it heals. Once we're born, that is. The fetus has the ability to heal without the formation of scar tissue. We do not. That is why there is so much research studying fetal wound repair. One of the goals of such is to identify children who will be born with cleft lips and palates and operate on the child in the womb, before it is born.

Even if you don't really see a scar, the scar tissue is there. Scars that

Figures 1–4: This patient, in her late thirties, complained about the lines that had formed over the last five years between her eyes and on her forehead.

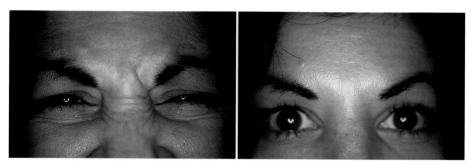

Figures 1 and 2: Before and after injection while attempting to frown. Often, patients make unusual expressions when strongly attempting to make an expression that they are physically unable to do. These are not expressions that are made during everyday life.

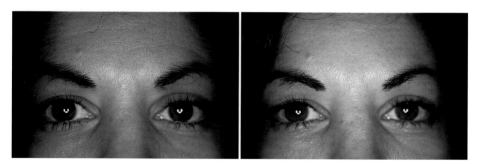

Figures 3 and 4: Note the tremendous improvement in her appearance while completely at rest. She has a slight bruise across the bridge of her nose. She had a high dose injected into this area due to the strength of these muscles, which really scrunched up her nose when she frowned (see upper left photo, Fig. 1). The horizontal wrinkles are gone from her nose and she was not left with the stigmata of the "Botox sign."

Figures 5–8: This young man in his thirties was not concerned about wrinkles or lines on his face. He felt his glowering appearance was affecting him negatively in the workplace.

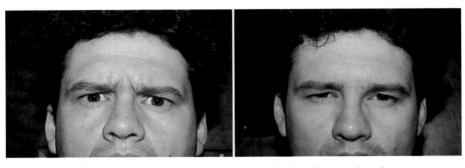

Figures 5 and 6: Frowning before and after injection. A standard result.

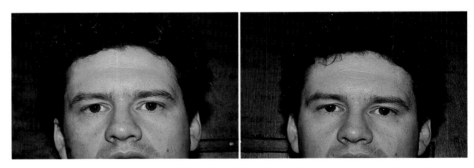

.Figures 7 and 8: What this patient liked best about his result was his appearance at rest. He lost his angry appearance and almost appears to be smiling (at least relative to the first picture) after treatment. If you cover the top part of the photo with your hand, you will see that there is no change in facial expression across his lower face. All of the improvement in his appearance is due to a simple Botox injection into his frowning muscles.

Figures 9–14: A woman in her fifties who was very concerned about her deep frown lines and moderate worry lines across her forehead.

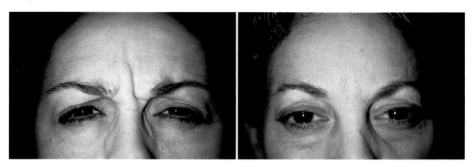

Figures 9 and 10: Frowning before and after injection. Obvious improvement.

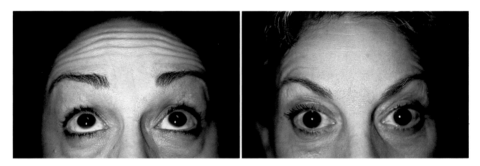

Figures 11 and 12: Raising eyebrows before and after. Forehead lines greatly improved despite good motion.

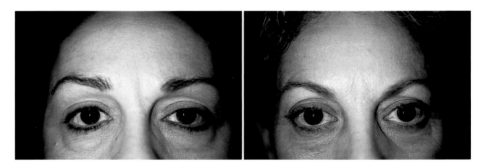

Figures 13 and 14: Dramatic improvement at rest. Her frown line was so deep that it could not be completely eliminated by Botox alone. If she wanted further improvement, a little collagen or other filler material in this area would be an excellent complementary treatment. Note the mildly droopy left upper eyelid before injection. This patient was at high risk for developing the dreaded eye droop after injection. This was recognized beforehand, and her injection pattern and dosage were changed accordingly. Not only did she not get an eyelid droop, but her slightly droopy lid actually improved!

Figures 15–32: This patient, in her late thirties, was primarily concerned about the position and shape of her brows as well as fine lines around her eyes, which were just beginning to show.

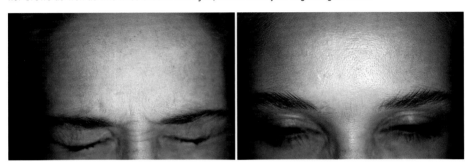

Figures 15 and 16: Maximal frown. Notice the near total lack of ability to pull her eyebrows near her nose in a downward direction.

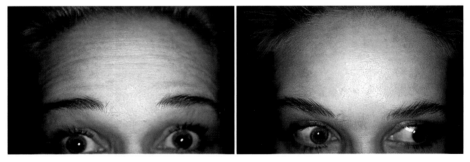

Figures 17 and 18: Raising eyebrows. Notice that before injection, this patient primarily raised her brows toward the center of her forehead, resulting in straighter, more masculine brows.

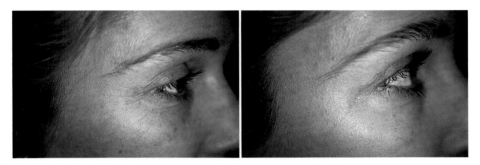

Figures 19 and 20: The outer right eye at rest. Notice the disappearance of her fine lines.

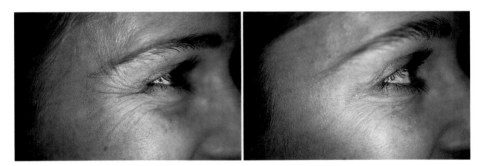

Figures 21 and 22: The patient is smiling. Notice the marked improvement, yet natural appearance. Even the small "roll" beneath her eye is improved.

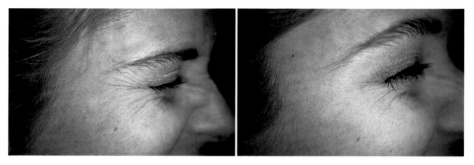

Figures 23 and 24: Squinting. With this increased effort, a smaller roll is seen beneath the eye.

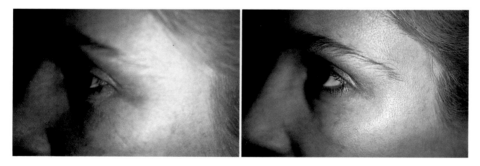

Figures 25 and 26: The left eye at rest. Fine lines begone!

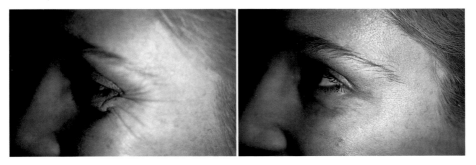

Figures 27 and 28: The left eye while smiling. The heaped-up skin at the edge of her lower eyelid is no longer there.

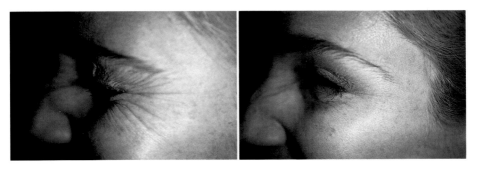

Figures 29 and 30: Full squint eye. Dramatic improvement.

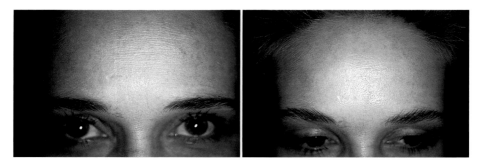

Figures 31 and 32: The patient at rest. I think this is the most important picture of the series. Her few wrinkles are gone despite her natural appearance and motion. The most important change for this patient, however, was in her brows. Before they were low, flat, and boyish. After, they are slightly elevated, curved, arched, and more feminine.

Figures 33 and 34: This patient in her late twenties was concerned about her heavy crow's feet lines and the hooding over her outer eyelid.

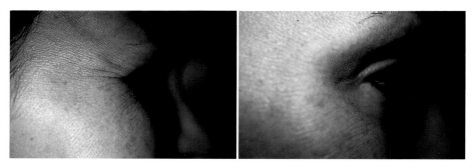

Squinting. Crow's feet and severe hooding are gone. Her eyelids are now visible.

are indented, discolored, in a straight line, and wide are usually fairly evident. Scars that are flat, the same shade as the surrounding skin, or thin and irregular are usually not. The goal of a scar revision is to turn a noticeable scar into a not-so-noticeable scar. "Erasing" scars can only happen before birth and in soap operas. I've done many scar revisions in my career. Basically, this involves sharply excising a scar, loosening up the surrounding skin by undermining it, and then bringing the skin edges together with sutures. Typically, scars from accidents heal poorly and are quite noticeable due to several factors. Obviously, most injuries do not occur under sterile conditions so some bacteria is introduced in the wound. Many cuts around the face are caused by a blunt force against the bone tearing the skin between them. When a cut is made in this way its healing is impaired. The reason for that is fairly simple. The edges of the skin, which need to heal together, have been crushed by the event that caused the cut. Since the skin has been crushed, its circulation and ability to heal will be impaired. Typically, a cut from a razor blade, broken glass, or other sharp object heals much better than a cut caused by blunt force. So, trying to revise a scar surgically usually improves the scar. That is because the repair is done with sterile instruments after preparing the skin with antibacterials. The scars are very sharply excised, taking care not to traumatize the skin left behind. But the third and I think most important step of a successful scar revision is to get the skin edges together with minimal tension. Tension across a wound causes an increase in the visible scar tissue. It is for that reason that Botox is very helpful when doing scar revisions on the face. With Botox, while the wound is healing, the muscles underneath it are not constantly pulling on the skin creating tension. What is truly interesting about Botox is its ability to make scars look better over years without doing any scar revisions or other therapy. Look at Figs. 93 and 94. This woman was injured in a car accident at the age of sixteen, resulting in scarring across both her frowning area and forehead. As expected, when I first injected her frowning area and forehead with Botox, not only her frown and worry lines got better but her scars were also less noticeable. This is because the scar was aligned in the wrinkles that she had already developed and motion appeared to make the scars actually worse. With the muscles no longer creating these motions the scars appeared flatter. This way the scars did not create an additional shadow drawing the eye toward them. But that was the expected result. What surprised me was comparing her pictures of several years apart. In these pictures, even though the patient is in the same state of partial weakness, the scarring appears much better four years later than it did previously. She is seen immediately prior to injection in both photographs. She had good motion when each picture was taken. I think that the Botox decreased the tension on the scar, and since scars are living tissue that remodel with time, the scar has become less noticeable without any additional treatment. Botox created, in essence, a revisionless scar revision.

The key to a good result in the forehead with Botox is to not overdo it. Just about anything—from Botox to collagen to a facelift to a nose job—looks bad when it is overdone. Except in the young patient with very fine lines, the goal in the forehead should not be to remove every wrinkle. A natural result occurs when you trade a little less expression for fewer lines and wrinkles.

See Crow's Feet Fly

The third area that I began to inject was the one just to the outside of the eye where crow's feet are formed. In 1991, this was a natural area for me to inject. You see, when I was a fellow at Manhattan Eye, Ear and Throat Hospital, one of the surgeons I studied under was Dr. Sherrell Aston. Dr. Aston had published a paper in the early 1980s describing a surgical technique to improve crow's feet. Each eye is surrounded by a circular muscle made of concentric rings radiating outward from the eye. The portion of this muscle that lies just to the outside of the eye, below the temple, is the part of the muscle that crinkles the skin in this area when we smile or squint. Dr. Aston had developed a surgical technique to weaken this muscle by surgically dividing it. The weakening of this small section of the muscle reduced the appearance of the crow's feet.

Well, if surgical weakening of the muscle improved the appearance of this area, I reasoned, so should Botox. So I began injecting the area outside the eye. The results were outstanding. In the younger patient early fine to moderate lines could be completely eliminated. Even the older patient with heavy lines and some excess hanging skin in this area had fair to good improvement.

In those early days, I frequently brought patients back about five days or so after their initial injection. I did this for two reasons. It is my personal philosophy regarding plastic surgery that you are much better off underdoing rather than overdoing something. So I would tend to inject a bit lightly in certain areas and then have the patient return a few days later to see the results. If the patient needed a little booster injection, I gave it at that time. The other reason I did this was because Botox was very expensive. I was very new to practice, and didn't have much money to waste. I knew that if I opened a bottle of Botox I could count on its working pretty well for at least a week. So, if the patient needed a little more, I wouldn't have to open a new vial just for a few drops. But the largest benefit of bringing patients back for a follow-up visit was in how it taught me to inject my patients more naturally. What really helped me was seeing nearly every patient that I injected just a few days later. That, coupled with practically living in the operating room and seeing the muscles I was injecting, really helped me discover the subtleties of proper Botox injection. I was learning quite a bit from my patients, and the idea was that I would inject them even better the next time.

One of the things that I gradually discovered is that the pattern of crow's feet was very different among different patients. If you think about it abstractly, you would suppose that everyone forms crow's feet in more or less the same way, with some people's wrinkles simply being worse than others. But not all crow's feet are created equal. People have very distinct crow's feet patterns. There are distinct patterns to muscular activity below the skin and thus the crow's feet pattern above the skin. The other thing I've learned in following these people over many years is that the patterns don't change with age. Advancing age may make the crow's feet deeper or more severe but it does not change their pattern. The most common pattern for crow's feet is what I call the full fan pattern. In these patients, the crow's feet start up top near the eyebrow, come down around the corner of the eye, and curl down into the upper cheek. Even though this is the most common pattern, it still occurs in less than 50 percent of the population. The next most common pattern has wrinkles starting at the corner of the eye but they are mostly limited to the lower eyelid and the area where the eyelid blends into the upper cheek. Patients with the third most common pattern primarily wrinkle the upper eyelid from the brow down to the corner of the eye. The least common pattern (only seen in 10 percent of the population) involves heavy wrinkling right at the corner of the eye but not much above or below it.

Another observation I made about crow's feet patterns was the lack of symmetry in some patients. In fact, 8 percent of patients have one wrinkling pattern outside one eye and a different pattern for the other eye. This asymmetry also does not seem to change with time. Most patients are not aware of small facial characteristics of their own that are asymmetrical. It helps to point this out to patients beforehand. If I don't, they will often scrutinize a recently injected area of their face and then think that I had created the asymmetry that had been there all long. Botox is an excellent tool for some patients with marked asymmetry who would like their face to be more symmetrical. By using different doses of Botox in the different sides of the face, asymmetry can be reduced. Asymmetry is not always a bad thing, however. An article was published many years ago in the plastic surgery literature examining the faces of people generally thought to be good-looking, including actors, models, and celebrities. Their faces were then split into mirror images. And all three views were shown: the face as it exists, the symmetrical face based on the mirror image of the left side, and a symmetrical face based on the mirror image of the right side. In every case the asymmetrical face was clearly more attractive. An argument could also be made from this study that people who are considered good-looking tend to be a little more asymmetrical than the population at large. I often do not try to correct every little asymmetry of the face that I see but that the patient hasn't noticed. Patients don't come to me so that I can make them *less* attractive.

Why should you care what pattern your crow's feet make? Because that pattern determines precisely how your Botox should be injected. Of all the areas that I have been injecting since 1991, I think I've changed my technique for crow's feet injection the most. A little while ago, I told you that I often eliminated crow's feet wrinkling in a great deal of my patients. I don't really like to do that anymore. I think that for a while I was overinjecting some people. If a person in her fifties is carrying on with a group of friends and laughing and smiling and there's not one crease in the skin next to the eyes, I think that looks unnatural and unattractive. Even teenagers, when beaming a big smile, have crow's feet. They are nothing to be ashamed of.

The woman whose crow's feet are seen in Figs. 19 through 30 was in her late thirties. This very attractive woman—like most attractive people—had a huge smile, and like most people with a great smile, lots of crow's feet. Fig. 19 shows a lot of early fine lines in the crow's feet area running down onto the lower cheek (another characteristic of people that we often find attractive). These lines are gone after Botox injection (Fig. 20). The next set of photos shows the patient smiling before and after injection in a full-fan-shaped pattern. Notice that in the after photo (Fig. 22) not only are the lines better, but she also does not pull her outer brow down as much. This reduces the hooding over her outer eye and lets you see more of her eyelid.

I also like to leave some crow's feet in place because of another observation that I have made over the years concerning good-looking people. If you were to study the faces of A-list actors (think Mel Gibson here), models (Lauren Hutton) and attractive celebrities (even Britney Spears) you would find that most of them actually have more crow's feet than most people the same age. On some faces, lots of crow's feet are actually attractive. My approach to the crow's feet during a consultation has changed greatly over the years. Usually, when patients come in for a Botox consultation, they have very specific areas in mind. Wrinkles in these areas have bothered them for years and they want them to be gone or at least made less noticeable. Most patients, however, sit in the chair opposite me and ask what I think we should do. Very often I'll recommend injecting the frown lines, worry lines, neck cords, chin dimpling, or smile lines. Then I tell them that I can decrease the appearance of their crow's feet lines in certain areas, which are pointed out to them in a mirror. I also tell them that some people look better with their crow's feet than without. Most patients do want their crow's feet to be reduced. But more and more people tell me that they "don't mind" their crow's feet. What they really mean is that they think their appearance is better with a little bit of crow's feet. I think that's the closest I'll ever come to hearing a patient tell me that they actually like wrinkles.

So why do very attractive people tend to have more crow's feet than the rest of us? Mostly because crow's feet come from smiling. Remember how dramatically Botox helped people with heavy frown lines. Even though these people were not angry, they were frequently perceived to be until Botox came along and removed that nasty look from their faces. It allowed these people to leave better first impressions and have better interpersonal relations almost immediately. Just as frown lines can make a negative first impression, smiling lines outside the eyes can create a positive impression. It tells the world that you are a happy, friendly, and outgoing kind of person. And that effect is not necessarily something you want to get rid of.

Another reason these people seem to be more attractive is the effect this area has on their smile. Just as there are different motion patterns for the muscle that creates the crow's feet, there are different smile patterns created by the myriad muscles that control how we smile. A classification of smile patterns was published in 1974 in the plastic surgery literature. The least common smile pattern, which occurs in only about 2 percent of the population, is the full denture, commonly called Hollywood smile. In this pattern, the smile is huge, revealing all of the upper teeth and a fair amount of the lower teeth as well. People with these large smiles are often considered attractive. While it occurs only in 2 percent of the population at large, in Hollywood I bet that figure is closer to 80 percent (think Julia Roberts or Tom Cruise). Most of the strong pull for this kind of smile comes from the muscles around the mouth. But in most people the little muscle that circles the eye contributes its share too. The lower outer portion of this muscle not only crinkles the skin next to the eye when we smile, it also helps to lift the upper cheek. So a portion of this muscle helps us to smile. If this portion of the muscle is completely weakened, the upper cheek will droop a bit and the smile will flatten. That is another reason to be conservative with Botox injections in this area. If you try to eliminate every wrinkle (except in patients thirty and under), you'll have an unnaturally smooth appearance and drooping of the upper cheek when smiling. Since this muscle helps to pull that upper cheek skin up, sometimes a little roll of skin is left on the border between the lower eyelid and cheek. This happens when the area is overinjected, because now the muscle can't lift the cheek skin up toward the corner of the eye as it's supposed to. The skin just sits there. So, when overinjected, the laughing patient not only has an unnatural flattened look to this area but the side of the face and upper cheek are actually drooping more than they normally would. It actually accelerates the aging process!

Let's go back to the patient we were just looking at. Her next two photos show her squinting (Figs. 23 and 24). Although the lines are better, she is still left with some motion, especially across the upper cheek, which contains the part of the muscle responsible for pulling up on the upper cheek. This allows her to still give her beaming smile. The next six photos show her other eye through the same progression: at rest, smiling, and squinting. These photos illustrate her asymmetry and corresponding change of injection strategy.

At rest (Figs. 25 and 26) her lines are gone. Smiling, she still has a full fan pattern to her wrinkling, but it is not as strong across her upper eyelid and brow while it is much stronger across her lower eyelid and upper cheek. When she smiles (Fig. 27), her left eye generates very few wrinkles above the corner of her eye but a large knuckle forms along her lower eyelid that was very unsightly, especially for such a youthful woman. Because of this, she received much less Botox to her upper lid on the left and a lot more to not only the lower crow's feet but right into the lower eyelid as well. This was something that the "experts" said should never be done. Her knuckle is gone and her lower lid is smooth (Fig. 28). Looking at her squinting photos (Figs. 29 and 30) her lines are better, almost too much better. I had to put so much Botox into her lower lid to get rid of her bump that the lower lid/upper cheek lines are a little weak on this side in Fig. 30. That is the trade-off for eliminating the bump.

The young patient in Figs. 33 and 34 also had tremendous improvement in her crow's feet lines. Since she was in her twenties, I had no qualms about injecting her strongly, eliminating her crow's feet even while squinting. This patient was pleased that both her wrinkles and the hooding effect of her upper eyelids was gone. She was unhappy about the fact that she could not leave her house without sunglasses on because she was extremely sensitive to light. She was always sensitive to light, but was able to block out most of it by squinting—this was why her crow's feet were so apparent in the first place.

Clearly, in the crow's feet area, too much of a good thing can have very undesirable results. In this area my average dose is less than half of what it used to be. In my mind, the unnatural deer-in-the-headlights look with a flat cheek and no lines outside the eye is extremely unattractive. So if less is more, how much weakening is good? I think that at least everyone from their late thirties to early forties looks better with at least some crow's feet when smiling. Conversely, I think that in almost any age patient, the appearance at rest is better without crow's feet. No crow's feet at rest, and present but not overpowering wrinkles during lively animation, is the perfect balance. It is a youthful balance. So how do I decide where to go light on the Botox? The answer lies in the crow's feet patterns.

If you looked at the anatomy of different patients' muscles around the eyes you would not see much variation. What you do have is a great degree of functional variation. What a patient's crow's feet pattern tells me is where that muscle is very active and strong and where it is relatively weak. It only makes sense to inject the overactive parts of the muscle that are responsible for most of the lines formed on the skin. This leaves the rest of the muscle to carry out its functions of closing the eye, supporting the lower eyelid, and helping to lift the cheek. This both reduces the unwanted lines *and* leaves the muscle functional.

I have no qualms about where I inject the areas of overactive muscle as long as the lower lid is taut and not in danger of falling away from the eye. I will even inject right up to the edge of the eyelid if that is where the overly dominant muscle is. For years many experts cautioned against this. I was in Turkey a few years ago injecting three patients on the stage before a large crowd of plastic surgeons and dermatologists. When I injected one patient right along the lower lid next to the eye I heard an audible gasp from the crowd. The moderator asked what I was doing. He said that you cannot inject that close to the eye. I asked him why. He said because Dr. So-and-so said so. I asked why again. He said because if you are that close to the eye, some Botox will seep into the muscles that control the eye's motion in the socket, leaving the patient with blurred vision. I asked him how many eyes he or his quoted expert had injected in this fashion. He replied none, of course. Who would want this complication? I then asked him if he knew how many eyes I had injected in this fashion. I didn't really know myself except that it was in the thousands. I then told him exactly how many patients I had given double vision to. The answer was—and is—zero. This is just another example of thinking of what *may* happen but not really paying attention to what *does* happen. Guess what happened a year or so later? Dr. So-and-so came out with a new, revolutionary, breathtaking paper saying that you can inject the eyelids close to the eye!

How much each patient will improve is very different. Remember, Botox is only working on the muscle. Eyelid skin is very delicate and is in a sun-exposed area of the face. The improvement here depends mostly upon the condition of the skin. If the skin has been damaged by years of sun exposure, smoking, or heavy drinking the improvement will be limited. In this case, the skin is often treated separately with either laser resurfacing or a chemical peel. Both of these treatments strip away the top layer of the skin, allowing new skin to heal in place from the bottom up. Unfortunately, deeper peels and laser resurfacing take ten days to two weeks to heal. During this healing period, Botox can work very synergistically with these procedures. The skin will heal more smoothly after resurfacing if it is not subjected to constant motion and crinkling. This is one situation in which I feel comfortable overinjecting a patient. If the result from laser resurfacing will be just a little better, I think it is worth it to have a slightly overdone look for a month or two.

This brings me back a bit to the often quoted "experts" who with each subsequent interview seem to have begun injecting Botox at progressively earlier dates. This is the case with someone recently quoted as saying she began using Botox years ago. I listened to her give a lecture a few months ago in which she said that she had a relatively new use for Botox. She said that we could now add Botox to our laser resurfacing treatment of this area since it would help the patient heal more smoothly. Nothing wrong with that. That is something everyone agrees on. But it's the little subtleties of language that sometimes raise questions. I've been using Botox in this area since 1991. This was years before laser resurfacing was a reality. Since Botox was then and is still now my first line treatment for crows feet for most patients, I added laser resurfacing to it. And that's how those of us who really have been injecting Botox since the early '90s say it. We didn't add Botox to our laser resurfacing, which came years later. We added laser resurfacing to it. A simple order of words that is very revealing.

Even if I think a patient's lines are primarily due to skin problems I will often try Botox before more aggressive skin resurfacing, due to the long healing time otherwise required. The Botox is sure to at least help a little and maybe a lot with the lines. If the result is less than spectacular, no bridges have been burned, and laser resurfacing is still an option.

This is an area where skin care has made a major difference. From Retin-A to glycolic acid to kinerase to vitamin C to microdermabrasion, these small "no downtime" procedures have a better overall effect when combined with Botox injections. Newer, less destructive lasers are also being used to treat the skin and require no healing time. While not as strikingly effective as the carbon dioxide or erbium lasers, the idea behind them is sound. They wound or damage the skin deeply, bypassing the superficial skin, which remains intact. This induces the deeper skin to contract, improving the appearance of the skin above. Presently, these machines do not give big results, but I believe they will as the technology moves forward.

When there is a lot of hanging skin outside the eye, the effect of Botox will be severely limited. This is another example of Botox working well with surgery. Eyelid surgery can remove the extra skin, allowing Botox to work its magic on the muscle below. Since this muscle circles the eye, a portion of it lies across the lower eyelid. This is also a good area to inject in certain people. Some will have fairly heavy horizontal lines immediately below their lower eyelid, not really outside the eye in the crow's feet area. A tiny bit of Botox in this area will go a long way to minimize the appearance of these lines. Care must be taken not to overinject this area also. The muscle in the lower eyelid actually has an important function. It holds the lower eyelid against the eye. In patients in their thirties and forties, this function is not so important, since the lower eyelid is usually fairly taut. But in some patients, the lower eyelid has been stretched and is fairly loose. In these patients only the muscle holds that lower eyelid up. Weakening this muscle in a patient with a loose lower lid can have disastrous results, with the eyelid actually falling away from the eye. Your injector should carefully evaluate your lower eyelid before injecting it.

I've occasionally had patients come to my office complaining of bags in their lower eyelid. Their appointment was made with me for surgical consultation. In most people, the bags are actually pockets of fat upon which the eyeball floats in the eye socket. They act as a sort of shock absorber for the eye. If the eye actually sat on the bone of the eye socket, every time your foot hit the floor while walking your vision would get blurry. Sometimes with time or even in a young patient this fat pushes against the inside of the lower eyelid and creates unsightly bulges on the outside. The bag can be surgically removed, resulting in a much smoother eyelid. But not all bags are fat. Sometimes, the bags that a patient complains about are actually a very thickened roll of muscle along the lower eyelid. In these cases, Botox can have outstanding results and eliminate the need for surgery. The patient in Figs. 95 and 96 had exactly this problem. When she came to my office for a surgical consultation, she pointed to the bags in her lower eyelids and said she wanted them removed. The thing was, her "bags" were not made of fat at all. She simply had an unusually large roll of muscle beneath the skin of her lower eyelid. Tiny drops of Botox were injected all along her lower eyelid, leaving just a thin strip of muscle working at the very top of the lid. This working muscle was enough to hold her lid up in a normal position. The large roll of muscle and her "bags" were gone. This was about seven years ago. She still has not had any eyelid surgery. One word of caution here: Overly weakening the muscle of the lower eyelid can sometimes let the fat behind it push out a bit more—actually creating "bags."

Injecting the lower eyelid itself (below the crow's feet area) can produce outstanding results to the patient with heavy wrinkles here. As opposed to crow's feet proper, almost nobody thinks that these lines look good. One word of caution about this area. When it is heavily injected, the lower lid will sag a bit. This exposes a little more of the eye. Sometimes this is touted as making your eyes bigger. But bigger is not always better. A sagging lower lid is also a sign of aging. Trying to make your eyes look bigger this way usually just makes them look older.

A major concern that many patients harbor prior to injecting this area is pain. The region around the eyes can be quite sensitive. This fear prevents many patients from trying Botox in this area despite the fact that they would have excellent results. In reality, of the three areas we've discussed so far, most patients agree that this is the least painful to inject because it requires a much more superficial injection. The muscles between the eyebrows and in the forehead are very deep just above the bone. The skin is fairly thick in these areas and the areas are filled with sensory nerves. Outside the eye, the muscle is very superficial. The skin is almost tissue-paper thin and there's very little fat between the skin and muscle. Since the injection is so superficial, there's very little pain associated with it.

In the mid-'90s, I used EMLA cream for a while to see if I could decrease the pain of Botox injections. EMLA, a cream that contains some local anesthetic, is applied to the skin about an hour before injection. It is frequently used in children. For several months, all my patients received EMLA prior to injection. I wasn't that impressed with the results. Then, the next fifty patients I saw in my office for Botox injections who had had at least one prior set of injections without EMLA and one set of injections with EMLA were questioned. They were asked if they wanted to use the EMLA before their injection. Only two out of the fifty thought it was worth the hour's wait. I have also used EMLA and some of the other anesthetic creams on myself in order to gauge their effect. Although the cream can dull or eliminate the pinprick sensation that your skin feels with a needle going in, that's not where most pain from a Botox injection comes from. Most of the pain comes from injecting the liquid into the muscle. These small ribbon-like muscles are each encased in a thin envelope, which is very inelastic. When the Botox is injected into the muscle there's no real room for it to go. That hurts. The problem with the anesthetic creams is that they only penetrate into the skin, making it numb so that you don't feel the initial pinch. But they don't penetrate all the way through this skin and through the fat almost down to the bone to where they can help with the pain in the muscle. The exception is in the crow's feet area. Since the skin is so thin and delicate there and the muscle is practically stuck right against it, the creams do have some effect here. Most patients I inject don't use the cream. The injections simply aren't that painful. But when I have a patient who is very needle-phobic, I recommend the cream for the crow's feet area especially.

Changing the Shape and Height of Your Brows

In recent years, eyebrows have rocketed to the top of the beauty obsession checklist. Nowadays, celebrity "eyebrow gurus" are the subject of many a fawning magazine profile, right alongside hairstylists, makeup artists, personal trainers—and plastic surgeons, of course. And just like the hot blush and lipstick shades, or the cool new 'do du jour, eyebrow trends from the runways are now eagerly anticipated each fashion season.

Of course, this isn't the first public go-round with brow fixation. In earlier decades, brows were a key element of the overall look for stars like Marlene Dietrich and Joan Crawford. But after a period when brows took a backseat, they're firmly back in the limelight. And there is no question that several of today's hottest properties have undergone fairly dramatic transformations from a well-wielded pair of tweezers. (Need proof? Just take a peek at a few mid-'90s shots of Madonna, Elizabeth Hurley, or Jennifer Aniston.)

If to today's beauty-savvy consumer, it's all about the brows, for doctors, however, it's all about the "peri-orbital" area of the face. Consisting of the eyeball, upper and lower eyelids, upper portion of the cheekbone and brow, this entire area is what I zero in on when patients come in for a "brow consultation."

As the cornerstone of attractiveness for the upper portion of the face, the peri-orbital area is of critical importance. And it has also, prior to the advent of Botox, been the focus of many a plastic surgery procedure. But while surgery can change—at least slightly—the apparent size and shape of the eye, that type of procedure does not have many points in its favor. Complex procedures like this can move the eyes closer together or farther apart, change the shape of the eye from round to almond, and sometimes even alter the apparent size of the eye relative to the surrounding structures. Not only is this surgery considered radical, its outcome is somewhat unpredictable and permanent. It is not a procedure with a great deal of inherent finesse. Given these drawbacks, not many people who want to change their look would opt for this. What is relatively malleable, however, is the brow. It is actually quite easy to change and, because it frames the eye, can dramatically improve appearance.

But how much do actual brow trends play into a consultation with a plastic surgeon? It depends on the patient. I would never advocate plastic surgery simply to achieve a stylish or trendy look. Surgery is a serious, long-term business. Near the opposite end of the serious spectrum is Botox. While Botox injections are not quite on the same level as having your hair cut, they only take about fifteen minutes and are not permanent. That's an advantage here; you can use Botox to achieve different looks by manipulating the brow.

Unfortunately, most physicians don't realize this. They fail to see the different trends in brows, and how different eyes and faces need to be framed by different brows. Clearly, one size does not fit all. Despite this fact, plastic surgery textbooks are notoriously filled with pictures of the all-purpose "perfect" brow look. In fact, I've seen geometric, mathematical drawings describing exactly the perfect length and curvature of the brows. While this may be helpful to a beginning plastic surgery student, or someone who has no eye for aesthetics, he/she is probably not the best bet to shape your brows with Botox in the first place.

While there is no ideal brow for everyone, there are obvious differences between men and women. In the old days, only women plucked and thinned their brows. No longer. Today, many men pluck, thin, and shape their brows. And some, like me, have brow-shaping thrust upon them by well-meaning beauty professionals. About a year ago, while I was having my hair cut, I was sitting peacefully in the chair with my eyes closed when all of a sudden I felt a tug and a snip along my right brow. Yikes! Obviously, I had no choice but to let the hairstylist work his magic on the left brow, as well. Of my first five thousand Botox patients, 16 percent were men—and almost all had some change in shape and position of their brows.

The positioning of the brow in general is also different between the sexes. Women tend to have a higher brow, situated slightly above the bone that forms the upper boundary of the eye socket. Man, perhaps befitting his more Neanderthal nature, has a lower, overhanging brow that is usually below the bone of the upper eye socket. While most men do have some curve toward the outside of the brow, it's certainly much less pronounced than in most women.

Just what type of brow-area impact can you expect from Botox? Although there is some disagreement within the aesthetic community, there are actually two aspects of brow shape that Botox can control very well: the height of the brow and the degree of curvature or shape of the brow.

Patients are often misinformed about the ability of Botox to raise, lower, and/or shape the brows. It's no wonder misconceptions abound; just as the popularity of Botox has exploded in recent years, so has the number of Botox "experts." With the rush of practitioners—from many fields, several of which are completely unrelated to aesthetic procedures—the amount of inaccurate information distributed to the public has been truly alarming. Oftentimes, it underscores pretty shocking ignorance not only of the potential effects of Botox but also of basic musculature and physiognomy.

Case in point: A few years ago, I was attending one of the two large annual plastic surgery conferences. A paper was presented concerning rejuvenation of the eye area. The lead author had previously presented a Botox paper that was based on over a thousand patients. Thus, one would assume that this person would be very knowledgeable about the effects of Botox on the eye area. However, the main "take-away" of this new paper was that since Botox only weakens the muscles, it can be used solely for the purpose of lowering the brows (or, at best, leaving them where they are). What this paper—and its author—failed to take sufficiently into account is that there are *several* muscles that actually function to pull the brows down. So when these muscles are injected with Botox, the brows spring up. Perhaps this author had skipped the same meeting of the previous year, at which I had presented my own paper detailing the ability of Botox to elevate the brows!

Not that raising the brows with Botox is as easy as it may sound. There are thirteen different muscle segments that can actually depress the brow. Not all of these muscles depress the brows in all patients. In addition, there's the forehead musculature, which raises the brows. All of these muscles are interactive, and in a very delicate way, control the shape and position of the brows. By partially weakening different portions of the different muscles, it's possible to raise the brows quite dramatically. You can also control where the brows are elevated. For example, I can raise each of the outer, inner, or middle portions of the brows. It's pretty extraordinary.

In fact, I've found that the control I have in shaping the brows is greater with Botox than with any surgical procedure.

But you don't have to take my word for it. Let's look at some examples. The woman in Figs. 15 through 32 is in her late thirties. As you can see in Fig. 31, she doesn't have much in the way of lines on her forehead or brow. Even when she is trying to wrinkle her brow and forehead, in Figs. 15 and 17, the wrinkles are pretty superficial. Two things stood out when I examined her: the crow's feet lines with a large muscle roll along the lower eyelids and her brows. If you study her brows in Fig 31, you can see that they are fairly low, just beneath the ridge of bone that forms the top of the eye socket. But they aren't just low, they are flat as well. Clearly she had tried tweezing the lower hairs along the outer portion of the brow in an attempt to give herself a bit of an arch, without much success. The problem is how flat the upper border of the brow appears.

You have to take everything into account when changing someone's brows. While her brows were somewhat masculine, she was still a very attractive woman. She was very athletic and had a tomboyish appeal. To attempt to really crank up her brows as high as possible would have been a mistake. A dramatic high, fine brow would have been out of place on this patient. So I decided—along with removing her crow's feet lines and that heaped-up knuckle of muscle on her lower lid—to gently arch her brows more toward the middle of the brow rather than just at the outer third and to gently raise the brows only a few millimeters.

The first step was to completely knock out the ability of the frowning muscles to pull down on her inner eyebrows. When you first look at the difference in Figs. 15 and 16, you'll notice that the frown lines are gone. But it's not just the frown lines. Those early horizontal lines along the bridge of the nose are gone too. Most people at this age don't make those horizontal lines as strongly as they make the vertical frown lines. This led me to believe that the muscles pulling down in this area were much stronger than in an average patient. Forget about the lines on her face for a second; now just look at where her inner eyebrows are positioned while making exactly the same expression in the two photos. They are much higher simply because the downward pull on them has been eliminated and they are farther apart.

But I didn't want this patient's brows to be too elevated. To prevent this I seriously weakened the center of her forehead. In Figs. 17 and 18, obviously the forehead lines are better. But that's old hat by now. Even a poor injector of Botox can make those lines less obvious. By weakening the center of her forehead, I dropped the inner portion of her brows back down but left the middle portion of the brows elevated. The forehead above the middle brow was not weakened. In addition to only desiring moderate brow elevation, I did not want an overly dramatic shape to the brow with the outer brow incredibly high. For this reason, I slightly weakened the outer forehead above the outer brow. I knew the outer brow would rise up a little anyway, since the crow's feet muscle had been severely weakened and was no longer pulling down on the outer eyebrows. This was the first time that I had ever seen this patient. In retrospect, I probably overinjected her forehead a bit. For subsequent injections, I decreased her forehead dose but did not change the pattern of my injections.

The most important photos of this series are Figs. 31 and 32. They show the patient in her natural, relaxed state. Her brows are slightly elevated but not overdone. While she did not have any wrinkles per se beforehand, her skin is much smoother. But the big difference is in the shape of her brows. Look at the line formed by the top of her eyebrows. It has gone from completely flat to a nice gentle curve. These photos were taken five days apart. No other treatment was given, no brows were plucked. This patient could have achieved some curving of the brow with aggressive plucking, but that would have left her with very thin, dramatic brows, which would not have fit in with her overall look.

The two patients in Figs. 35 through 38 illustrate how Botox can give you control over different segments of the brow. Both before- and after-photos show the patients at rest. Both patients had previously tweezed the lower, outer portion of the brow to give it the appearance of being arched and lifted, with different degrees of success. The first patient (Figs. 35 and 36) was not happy about the position of her outer brow.

She wanted it higher. This person has sharp, angular, attractive facial features and she wanted a more dramatic appearance. What really bothered her wasn't her brows directly. Over the last year or two she had noticed a little extra roll of skin at the very top of her eyelids, just below the bone above her eye. This patient requested two things: Botox for her forehead and brows as well as upper eyelid surgery to remove the excess skin from her upper lid. "Excess" as it refers to skin is a relative term. What it really means is excess skin to cover a designated area. In this case, that area is from the brows to the edge of the upper eyelid. So, surgery would decrease the amount of skin to cover this area, eliminating the excess. But if I could raise her outer eyebrows enough (the roll of skin was only visible under the outer brows), there would be a greater area for this skin to cover, also eliminating the excess. So I told this patient not to schedule surgery, that we'd see how much lift I could give her with just Botox, and if it wasn't enough, we could always do the surgery later.

Her after-picture tells the rest of the story. Her skin is smoother. The lines across the middle of her forehead are gone, since I strongly injected the middle of her forehead. Nothing happens in the human body without the body's reacting. Here, since the middle of the forehead was very weak, the outer forehead tried to compensate for it and pulled up even harder. This reaction alone lifted her outer brows about one-quarter of an inch. That may not sound like a lot, but when it comes to brows it certainly is. She did not have her crow's feet area injected. All of the outer brow lift that you see here was caused by inducing the outer forehead to pull harder on the brows. Another idea that I hear presented at medical meetings is that maybe you can get a tiny lifting of the brows initially but that it is very short lived and decreases with subsequent injections. I disagree with that completely. You can see with her brows up that the extra roll of skin that she wanted cut out is gone. These pictures are over six years old. This patient is still in my practice and I still have not had to surgically remove that skin.

The next patient (Figs. 37 and 38) had the opposite problem. She liked how tweezing the outer brow brought that portion of the brow above the bone. But she didn't like how her inner brows now seemed low by comparison. This patient, unlike the last one, has a heart-shaped face with softer features. An overly high dramatically arched brow did not look good on her. This was an easy one. I completely paralyzed all of the muscles that pulled down on her inner brows. This gave her a slight brow lift limited to her inner brows only.

The woman in Figs. 39 through 42 shows a different and more frequently desired type of result. This attractive woman has huge, bright blue eyes that dominate her face. She also shows (Fig. 41) a lot of her upper eyelid. This look was commonly referred to in the '50s as "bedroom eyes." While she liked her eyes, she did not like how her brows seemed to crowd them by hanging a bit low. They were not doing a very good job of framing her big beautiful eyes. Her case was complicated by another matter. When she was a teenager, her left eyelid was noticeably lower than her right. She also started to develop horizontal wrinkles across her forehead in her early twenties. I figured this happened because her forehead was desperately trying to help her eyelid muscles lift her eyelids up a bit more. All this activity had prematurely aged her forehead.

So I had to raise her eyebrows but I also wanted to weaken her eyebrow-raising muscles to improve her forehead's worry lines. What I did was weaken her forehead everywhere except directly over her brows. I also completely paralyzed all thirteen muscle segments that could pull down on her brows. In Figs. 39 and 40, you can see her raising her brows before and after her injections. She still has a lot of motion, although she cannot lift her inner brows very much, for that we would depend on the lack of a downward pull from her brow depressors. Even during motion, her forehead lines are gone.

Her at-rest pictures (Figs. 41 and 42) tell the story. Her lines are gone. Her brows are lifted all over. Even if you were to just look at her inner brows, they have gone from resting beneath the bone that frames the eye socket to sitting on top of it. The middle and outer brows are raised even more. As befits someone with this facial structure, the arch of the brows has also been increased.

Ultimately, success depends on understanding how all these different

muscle segments affect the brow. Sometimes patients don't fully understand the process, and, midprocedure, will question why I'm injecting
their upper eyelid, the bridge of their nose, or the middle or outside of
their forehead rather than directly into the brow. The answer? That's
where the muscles that pull, raise, lower, and change the shape of the
brow reside. Very rarely are the brows themselves directly injected.

The degree of control I can achieve with Botox over brow shape and
position is precise—considerably more than can be achieved with surgery.
As a result, I've noticed a marked decrease in the annual number of surgical forehead and browlifts. By now I think most plastic surgeons across
the country would agree that the number of surgical fixes for these two areas is in decline. And the reason is Botox. In the early '90s, when physicians would ask me about the primary uses of Botox, I would recommend
it as a precursor to a full-blown surgical browlift. During the latter procedure, the muscles that wrinkle the brow and give us worry lines are surgically removed and thrown away. The permanence of this procedure would
obviously give some patients pause. "What would that look like?" they
would ask. "What would it feel like not to be able to frown?"

So I would let them see for themselves. I would inject them with
Botox a few months before their surgery, which would give them some
idea of the potential result. And that continued to be a good use of
Botox in my practice for several years. Then I had an idea: in the late
'90s, I was invited to give a speech on Botox. And as a matter of habit,
because there's always a chance that audience members have heard me
speak on the topic of Botox before, I always try to introduce new material
into my talks. So I decided to look through my patient photographs and
pull those who had been injected with Botox as a preview of brow surgery. I would then show their before- and after-surgery pictures as well.
It was a good idea but it didn't work. Why? Because no one who had
been given the Botox preview had ever gone through with their scheduled browlift surgery. If I had a patient who had been booked for a
facelift, upper and lower eyelid surgery, rhinoplasty, chin implant, and
browlift, and that patient had a Botox preview, he or she opted for
everything but the browlift.

This is not to say that Botox does exactly what a browlift does. And while most patients have an excellent result with a Botox browlift, not everyone does. The patient with very low brows and heavy horizontal wrinkles in her forehead will have a hard time achieving more than a mediocre result with Botox. That's because the horizontal lines of the forehead are caused by the eyebrow-lifting muscles, which must be weakened. Sometimes, however, a little weakening is a good thing for brow-positioning. When one portion of the eyebrow-lifting muscles is weakened, the other positions usually pull harder to try to compensate. In that way, you can really raise part of the brow while depressing other parts of the brow and arching the brow tremendously. While not completely replacing the surgical browlift, there's enough overlap and gray area between the two so that Botox can certainly replace many browlifts and easily delay others for several years.

Laugh Lines Got You Down?

While I was still a fellow at the Manhattan Eye, Ear and Throat Hospital, I traveled to Los Angeles for one of the two large annual plastic surgery meetings. I was there to present the paper that I had written along with Dr. Lisman. While there, I heard many new papers and presentations being given. Some were good, some not so good. But one was outstanding. This paper was presented by Dr. Joel Pessa. The paper was about the laugh lines that run from our nostrils down to around the corners of our mouths. Dr. Pessa tried to determine which muscles were primarily responsible for these lines. Several different factors converge to give us these lines. One of the most important is the musculature in this area of the face. The muscles that produce a smile are actually attached to the undersurface of the skin along the laugh lines. When these muscles contract, they pull up on the undersurface of the skin, allowing us to smile but also creating an indentation. The precise goal of the paper was to determine the relative contribution of each of the muscles of facial expression in this area that create the laugh lines.

There is one muscle in particular, the muscle closest to the nose, that disproportionately causes a great deal of the laugh lines and only very minimally affects the smile. Its name is the *Levator Labii Superioris Alequae Nasii* muscle. For obvious reasons, I like to abbreviate the name and call it the LAN muscle. Dr. Joel Pessa embarked on a study in which some patients had the LAN muscle surgically divided and permanently weakened. That scared me a little. I was still a fellow and just about to start my private practice, and I was a bit too conservative in nature to permanently weaken some people's faces. But I thought it would be a great area to try some Botox. If it worked, great. If the results were not so good, the effects would go away in a few months.

In May 1992 I began to inject the LAN muscle with Botox. I started with very small doses and gradually increased the amount until I saw a result. The results were encouraging. I looked back at my first few dozen patients to see if the results were really as good as I thought they were. Of these patients, about two-thirds were pleased enough with their results to return for another injection. In today's environment, this would not be a very scientifically sound way to determine if patients were happy with their result. Where my practice is located, there is literally someone injecting Botox on every corner. So these patients can very often go from doctor to doctor. But in 1992 I think it is safe to say that I was the only doctor doing this. So most of my patients were satisfied but not enough for me to be satisfied. The patients who were unhappy all had the same complaint. When they smiled, their upper lip did not raise as high after the injection as it did before. So they were showing less of their upper teeth and consequently appeared to have less of a smile. That is because even though the LAN muscle mostly creates the laugh lines, it also contributes a small amount to lip elevation. Certain patients were more unhappy than others with this technique. If the patients naturally tended to only show a small portion of their upper teeth when smiling before injection, they showed no teeth after the injection. The result was a sort of strange, toothless grin. But to me, this procedure still made a lot of sense. It was based on very sound principles. The problem was with patient selection. It should come as no surprise that not everyone smiles

the same way. Just as with the crow's feet lines, there are certain rec-
ognizable smile-line patterns in patients. The most common pattern is
what is commonly referred to as the Mona Lisa smile. In this smile the
muscle called the *zygomaticus major* is the dominant muscle. This muscle predominately raises the corners of the mouth. So, in this most common type of smile, the strongest, most dominant feature is the corners
of the mouth turning up. The next most common type of smile is called
the canine smile. In this smile, the predominant muscles reside above
the middle portion of the upper lip. When these patients smile, they are
predominately raising the central upper lip as well as corners of the
mouth. Thirty-five percent of the population has this smile pattern.

Figs 55 and 56 show someone with a classic Mona Lisa smile before
and after injection. During her normal smile, she primarily raises the
corners of her mouth. After injection she still is primarily raising the
corners of her mouth but it appears more exaggerated. That is because
the LAN muscle helps to pull up the middle of the upper lip, which has
drooped a bit in Fig. 56. What is also readily apparent is that the smile
lines close to the nose are almost completely gone. All that remain are
the shorter lines around the corners of the mouth.

Since canine smilers tend to raise the middle portion of their upper
lip when smiling, I thought they would be excellent candidates for the
LAN muscle injection. These patients can usually afford to lose a little
raising of their upper lip. In fact, I thought that even without the
smoothing of the smile lines, some patients would actually look better
just from not raising the upper lip so severely. So I began to limit my
injections to this third of the population. Not surprisingly, my results
were a lot better. A lot of the patients did like their smile better after it
was converted into the more common Mona Lisa smile pattern with
Botox. But not everyone. Before injecting this area, I spend a bit of time
going over the risks and benefits with patients. I tell them that although
they are candidates for the procedure, it is definitely not for everyone.
While some people love the results and regularly have this area injected,
some do not. And it does not have to do with objective results. Case in
point: when I was going through my photographs for this book, I found

a set that I considered my best smile line before-and-after set. This set of photographs does not appear in this book. Why? Because although I objectively thought the patient's result was outstanding, she hated it, became angry, and so did not give her permission to use them. How we look when we smile is deeply ingrained in our minds. To change that look can really throw some people off. And it can affect the people around them. Just as common as hearing "I just didn't like it" was "I really liked the way it smoothed out my lines but my husband thought it made me look too different." Other uses of Botox that we've gone over basically involve reducing lines (that did not used to be there) and raising eyebrows (back to where they used to be). These are not big changes in our mind's eye. In fact, due to our selective memories, it often helps us to look more like our mental images of ourselves, which tend to be more favorable than reality.

Figs. 57 and 58 show someone with a canine smile before and after injection. If you compare her before picture to 55 you will see the difference between a canine and a Mona Lisa smile. The canine smile shows more of the upper teeth. The central portion of her upper lip is the highest part of her smile. The raised upper lip and not the corners of the mouth dominate this smile. Since these muscle dominate, it makes sense that the upper smile lines closest to her nose are deeper than those in the patient in 55, even though the patient in 57 is a decade younger. The improvement seen in the smile lines in 58 is dramatic, yet she still has a nice smile. While she liked her result, she said that family members thought she looked too different.

Although not a classically described smile pattern in the plastic surgery literature, I think the gummy smile should have its own categorization. In this type of smile, the middle portion of the upper lip is raised so severely that patients not only show all of their upper teeth but also some of their upper gums. To my mind it is sort of an extreme version of the canine smile. Most patients with this type of smile don't like it. They often find themselves covering their mouth with their hand when they smile or trying to force themselves not to smile so hard. Going hand-in-hand with the gummy smile are severe laugh lines especially close to the nose. This makes sense. Gummy smilers are people that tend to have overly expressive faces. In chapter 7, Making It Last, I will discuss which patients tend to get long-term results and which don't. Patients with extremely animated or almost cartoonish faces tend to not get long-term results, which is also the case for patients with gummy smiles. Since the smile lines are only slightly weakened, the effect does not last very long. Early on, I tell patients to expect only about six to eight weeks of results. Afer several injections, the results last closer to three months, perfect because these patients tend to come back about every three months for the rest of their face, anyway.

Patients with gummy smiles have LAN muscles that pull so hard that they raise the lip above the level of the gum. When a muscle pulls that hard it usually makes a rather severe wrinkle. Something else I've observed in these patients over the years is that their smiles are frequently asymmetrical. That is, one LAN muscle is pulling even harder than its counterpart, which is pulling pretty hard to begin with. These patients have outstanding results with Botox injections to their LAN muscles. The side with the stronger muscle gets a higher dose. This does several things. Their smile is no longer so crooked, their smile no longer reveals their gums, and their laugh lines are noticeably smoother.

The patient in Figs. 59 and 60 illustrates this very well. She has a gummy smile that is asymmetrical. She raises her right upper lip (on your left) much more strongly than her left. When I first started to inject her about five years ago, she needed a few touch-up injections to get everything just right. In her after photo her smile is less severe, more symmetrical, and her smile lines have gone from sharp dents to smooth grooves. She is extremely happy with her results and comes back regularly every three to four months for reinjection.

Figuring out how much of a higher dose to put in the stronger side sometimes takes a little fiddling. The first time I inject someone in this area I schedule a follow-up appointment for one to two weeks later. Even though initial effects of the Botox become evident in two or three days, sometimes it takes one to two weeks for all of the noninjected muscles to react to the weakened muscles and find a new balance. The touch-up rate for this area initially is high. I estimate that I need to inject a little more in either both or one side about one-fourth of the time. Sometimes a little asymmetry is revealed after weakening both muscles the same and sometimes I just underestimate the dose. But that is fine. I would much, much, much rather underestimate the dose and have the patients come back to the office for a little more than overinject and have them walking around with their upper lip hanging down looking like Cornelius from *Planet of the Apes.* For subsequent injections, once I have an individual's dose down, touch-ups are rare.

What surprised me initially was how much smoother patients looked even when they were not smiling or laughing. Certainly there is a resting tone in all the muscles of the body, but I was surprised by how much resting tone there was in the LAN muscle. Whenever evaluating Botox results in any area, it is important to see the patient both in animation and in repose. I remember presenting my work with smile lines at the American Society for Aesthetic Plastic Surgery meeting in Dallas in 1999. The presenter before me showed patients only at rest in the before and after examples. The presenter after me showed patients only in extreme animation. Both were, in my opinion, ridiculous. I have seen enough strange Botox injections to know that sometimes a patient will look great in animation and absolutely terrible in repose and vice versa. I would have loved to show you every set of photographs in this book in full animation and repose but due to space limitations that would be impossible. I have included both stages of animation where I felt it was absolutely necessary.

For the next patient, in Figs. 61 through 64, shots while smiling and in repose are included. This patient has a classic, mildly asymmetrical, gummy smile. During our consultation, she told me she wanted me to inject her wherever I thought it would be good. I cautiously brought up the smile line area and was going into my disclaimer about how it would change her smile. That's when her face brightened and she said, "I hate my smile." In Figs. 63 and 64 you can see that she no longer shows her gums when she smiles, and her smile lines look like those of someone in her mid twenties (she is thirty-nine). Even at rest her smile lines are much improved, especially close to the nose. This patient had no other treatment. No collagen or other fillers were used.

Injecting the smile area is not for everyone. In my practice it is limited to the 35 percent of us who have a classic canine smile. However, even some of these patients don't like the result. They want to look better, not change their appearance. People often identify themselves with their smile even if they're not crazy about it. Looking in the mirror and smiling and not seeing the same smile they've seen all their life can be a bit jarring.

Botox injections for the smile lines have gotten a bad rap for several reasons. One, some experts have taught other doctors to inject Botox into the *zygomaticus major* muscle. This is the muscle that lets us smile. Patients don't like not being able to smile. Two, patients were improperly selected (this is not for everyone). Three, even in good candidates it is easy to overinject this area. Four, even patients with good objective results sometimes do not like the change in their appearance.

Not only are the 35 percent of us who are canine smilers potential candidates for the injection but also the 5 to 10 percent of us who are gummy smilers are outstanding candidates for injection. I can't tell you have many times a patient has been to my office for the first time and when I told her that this was an area Botox could work for her she responded by saying Dr. So-and-so said that you can't use it in the smile lines. The most common response when asked why not is that it makes it so that you cannot smile and you look terrible. Everyone in my photographs can smile. That being said, Botox is not my most common treatment for the smile lines. That is because smile lines are created by many causes, not just the action of muscles. As we age, the skin tends to stretch and hang over the smile lines so that there is true excess of skin in this area. Also, the fat beneath our skin tends to slide down and in toward our mouths. But the fat can't slide past the smile lines. If you look at someone who's one hundred, the person doesn't have puffy, fat upper lips. The fat doesn't slide down that far. The fat is stopped at the smile line from descending any farther. That is because since the muscles that allow us to smile are attached to the underside of the skin along the smile line, this creates a pocket past which the fat cannot go. So the smile lines are also created by the fact that in many people there is an abundance of fat that you can easily pinch between your fingers above the laugh lines (try it now on yourself) but very little fat below the smile lines. And this mound of fat immediately above the smile line tends to emphasize the valley immediately below it. A fourth factor also contributes to the lines. A few years later, Dr. Pessa presented another study dealing with the smile lines. By reviewing CT scans of random patients at different ages, he found that as we age, our bones actually recede in this area. One more pleasant thought to send you off to sleep tonight. So, the smile lines are caused by excess hanging skin above, a sharp transition line between having a lot of fat above and very little fat below, the action of the smiling muscles pulling on the skin, and an actual deepening depression in the bone that supports this area as we age. How much improvement you can get from a Botox injection there depends on how much the lines are due to muscular action and not the other three factors. So if someone had a canine or even a gummy smile, if the person were old enough to have excess hanging skin over the fold, I wouldn't inject that person. You wouldn't see that much of an improvement in the smile lines but you would still see the slight drooping of the upper lip.

Because of these different causes, my most common treatment for smile lines is the injection of filler material, either collagen or fat. This helps to ease the transition between a lot of fat above and just a little fat below. It also helps to fill in the little groove along the line. Of course, this is not the ideal treatment for this area. The ideal treatment would be a surgical procedure that lifts and removes the excess skin, lifts the fat (which has slid down to the pocket just above the smile lines), and replaces it over the cheekbones where it used to be, and inserts an implant or filler material to build back up the deepening groove in the bone. With these three areas addressed, a little Botox to weaken the muscular contribution to this line would be the final touch. But that's a surgical procedure, and most patients are willing to settle for the smaller quick fix until the they start to receive diminishing returns. I don't want to mislead you; even a facelift doesn't get rid of the smile lines. Even though the skin and fat have been addressed, muscles are still pulling on that skin, creating a line. But that's okay. Most people have smile lines from their early thirties on. Not having a smile line at all would look very strange. In fact, the only patients I ever see without smile lines are those who suffer from Bell's palsy or a traumatic event that paralyzed half of their face. Even though the paralyzed half looks strange and droops and hangs since it no longer has muscular support, if you were to just look at the smile line area, it would appear much smoother than on the normal side of the face. I often tell some of my more demanding patients that the only people who don't have smile lines are people whose faces have been paralyzed.

Botox for the Chin and Lips

Perhaps the biggest misconception about Botox is that it really works well only for the upper face. I have been to many national meetings and heard many speakers I admire say that Botox has raised the bar so much for the upper face that we need to find something comparable to help us rejuvenate the lower face. Well, that something is Botox. Granted, it is a little trickier to use in the lower face, but in the properly selected patient, the results are outstanding.

Different people have different ways of expressing themselves. Besides language, people use their faces to communicate with others. Some people frown or will raise their eyebrows not to express anger or surprise but to command attention while speaking. In the same manner, some people jut their chin forward when making a point. Over the years, these people tend to ball up their chin, wrinkling it. Sometimes the skin over the chin gets a pattern that resembles a small waffle iron; sometimes it looks more like the dimples on a golf ball. However it looks, most of these patients wish that it just appeared smooth again. But chin-jutting is a difficult habit to break. Sometimes patients wrinkle their chin just while verbalizing certain sounds. These chin muscles are responsible for pushing our lower lip up against the upper lip. Some people make these patterns every time they chew their food, pushing the lower lip up, helping to seal the mouth.

Over years of exercising this otherwise relatively small muscle in the chin, it can become quite large and strong. In fact, after years of "working out" in this way, the skin starts to have a permanently dimpled appearance, even when the person isn't speaking. Before Botox, there was not a very good treatment for this condition. The lines are so small and irregular that injecting them with filler materials wouldn't produce a very good result. People would sometimes undergo dermabrasion or chemical peels, which involved a long recovery for only a small improvement. While these procedures could smooth out the skin a bit, the main problem, the muscles beneath the skin, was not addressed. During dermabrasion, anesthesia prevents you from feeling pain. But it is not the most fun recovery: you look as if you just walked off the set of a horror movie. In fact when I do a facelift, I often address the lines around the mouth with dermabrasion or laser resurfacing. Most patients tell me that the discomfort from the dermabrasion is worse than that from the entire facelift. It usually takes about two weeks just for the skin to reform, and it stays red for several weeks after that. In my practice, Botox has revolutionized treatment of these lines. The only time I recommend dermabrasion, deep chemical peeling, or laser resurfacing for this area is when someone is having another procedure at the same time (like a facelift) which would necessitate their hiding out for at least two weeks anyway.

Botox works so well on the the chin because of anatomy. The large, strong muscle that starts from the bone along the chin and goes up to the lower lip is firmly attached to the skin above it. There are strong fibrous attachments between the skin and muscle over the chin. So, when the muscle wrinkles, that wrinkle is directly transferred to the skin above it. If the Botox is simply injected into the bulk of this muscle or at the bottom of it where it gets its support from the chin, severe problems could result. Remember, this is the muscle responsible for holding the lower lip up against the upper lip. If you weren't able to do this, you wouldn't be able to seal your mouth and you wouldn't be able to drink fluids. You would drool. The key is to weaken only the superficial part of the muscle. That way the deep part of the muscle stays strong and is able to carry out its crucial function. But now the superficial part of the muscle will be relaxed and smooth, along with the skin above it. And the cobblestone pattern is no more.

A good example of this is seen in Figs. 75 through 78. These four photos are of the same patient. In Figs. 75 and 76 the patient is seen balling up her chin. She did this as a matter of habit during speech. Even when she was not talking but was resting with her mouth closed (Fig. 77) this cobblestoning or dimpling was present. When she was animated, besides the dimpling, it seemed as though she had a large block of something beneath her chin with shadows going around it. This was actually the block of muscle under her chin that had grown quite large over the years due to its constant use. When trying to ball up her chin after injection, she can neither make the dimpling appear nor does she look as though she has a knob on her chin. The clear borders along the outside of this muscle that created shadows and indentations are gone. The muscle now blends smoothly into the chin. Even at rest her appearance is clearly improved.

The area between the corners of the mouth and chin is also excellent for Botox. Here many patients begin to develop what are referred to as marionette's lines (think of Pinocchio with his wooden block of a chin and lower lip combined sliding up and down during speech and you get the picture). These lines run from the corners of the mouth down both sides of the chin. You can make these lines stand out on yourself by looking into a mirror and showing yourself your lower teeth. These are lines you probably make while you are brushing your teeth. As with the smile lines, there are many reasons these grooves are created. They form because the skin gets stretched and starts to hang over that line. And they form because the skin and fat get pulled down by gravity just outside this line, making it appear even deeper. And they form because a muscle runs beneath the line. This muscle's job is to pull down the corners of your mouth. Sometimes it is also somewhat adherent to the skin above it along its length and not just at the corners of the mouth.

Figures 35 and 36: This forty-year-old patient complained about the wrinkles on her forehead and frown lines, her low, flat eyebrows, and the fold of extra skin along her upper eyelid.

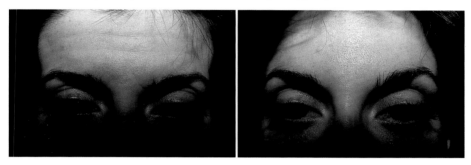

In repose before and after Botox injection to her frowning muscles and the central portion of her forehead. Her lines are gone and the outer portion of her forehead is now pulling her outer eyebrows up even harder. The apparent excess roll of skin at the top of the upper eyelid is gone since the eyebrows have been lifted over the outer portion of the eyes.

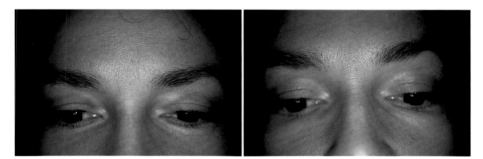

Figures 37 and 38: The patient above had an almost opposite request. She thought that her outer eyebrows were fine, but she wanted her inner brows lifted. Here the muscles that pull down on the inner brow have been completely paralyzed, allowing that portion of the brow to spring up.

Figures 39-42: This thirty-year-old patient was primarily concerned with the horizontal lines on her forehead that began to appear in her early twenties. She was also unhappy with her eyebrows, which were beginning to droop.

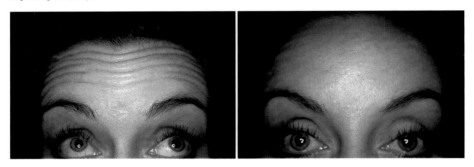

Figures 39 and 40: Raising eyebrows before and after. Normal expression seen.

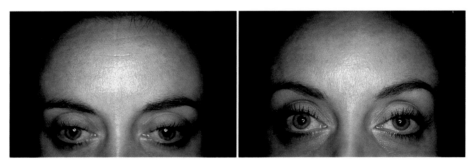

Figures 41 and 42: Obvious improvement of the fine, early wrinkles this patient was forming on her forehead and brow area. Note the elevation and increased arching of the brows.

Figures 43-46: The patient in the four photos below is in her fifties. She has a unique problem and had injections tailored to her anatomy.

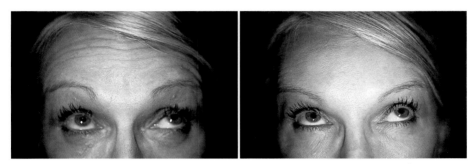

Figures 43 and 44: Raising brows. I injected her asymmetrically to induce her left eyebrow to pull up more strongly.

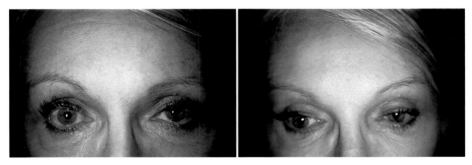

Figures 45 and 46: Not only does she look more refreshed and smooth, but her left eyelid and brow, which had been lower and flatter, have been raised and arched. This patient was also predisposed to develop a droopy eyelid, but with an individualized injection pattern that was avoided.

Figures 47–50: My own pictures. The author, in his late thirties, was concerned about the heavy frown line on his left side, which was more pronounced than on the right, as well as his heavy, low-set brows.

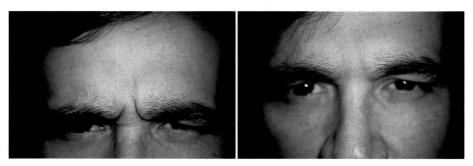

Figures 47 and 48: Frowning before and after injection. As you can see, I like to leave myself with very natural motion. I use the same technique for on-camera performers.

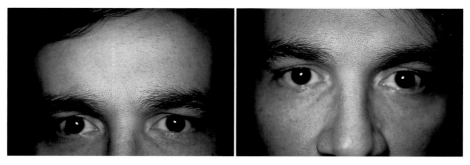

Figures 49 and 50: At rest. Notice the slight raising of my eyebrows so that you can see my eyelid all the way across. The brows are not overly arched or feminized.

Figures 51–54: This man in his mid-sixties was bothered by his frown lines, which made him appear angry, and by the hooding over the outside of his eyes when smiling.

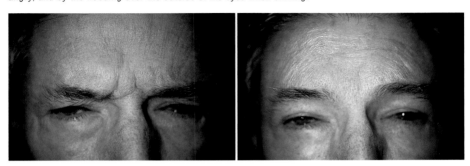

Figures 51 and 52: Frowning before and after injection.

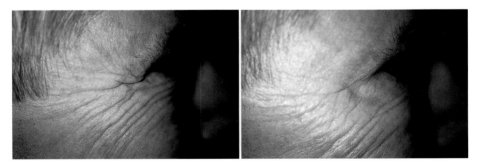

Figures 53 and 54: Smiling before and after crow's feet injection. Primarily his upper crow's feet were injected so that he would stop pulling down on his eyebrows and upper eyelids when smiling. I left him with some lower crow's feet to maintain a natural appearance and to avoid flattening of his smile.

Figures 55–58: The patients below had their smile lines injected.

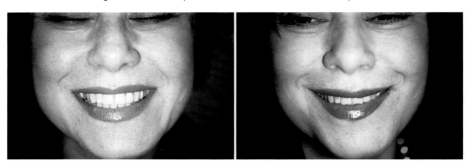

Figures 55 and 56: This patient has a classic Mona Lisa smile. Although her smile lines were markedly improved close to her nose, she was disappointed with the change in her smile.

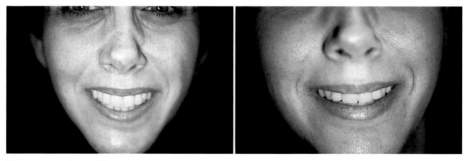

Figures 57 and 58: This patient has a more "canine" smile and thus a better result. Notice how smooth her smile lines are by the nose.

Figures 59-64: The two patients below are both excellent candidates for smile line injection.

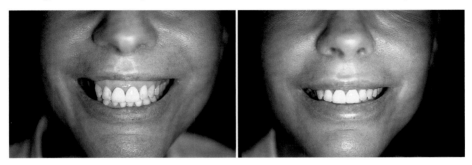

Figures 59 and 60: Before injection, this woman in her forties had a very asymmetric, gummy smile with sharp laugh lines. After injection, the laugh lines are smoother, her smile is straight, and her gums are not visible.

Figures 61–64: The patient below has a less severe gummy smile.

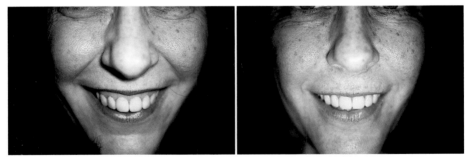

Figures 61 and 62: Photos of her smiling reveal less gum and tremendous improvement of her smile lines.

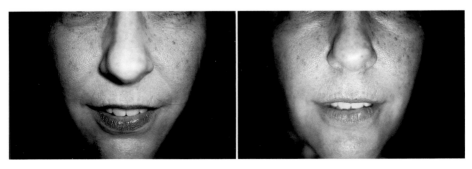

Figures 63 and 64: Even at rest, her smile lines are markedly improved despite her natural appearance.

Figures 65–68: This patient in her fifties complained of excess dimpling of both cheeks upon smiling.

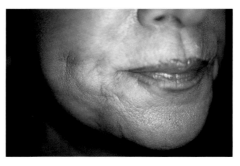

Figure 65: The dimpling of her right cheek prior to injection.

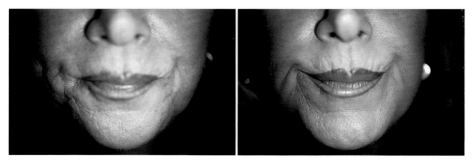

Figures 66 and 67: The above photos show the dimpling from a frontal view before and after Botox injection. Note the absence of extra lines around the corners of the mouth and cheeks.

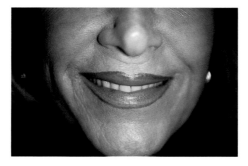

Figure 68: Completely normal, natural smile after injection.

If that is the case, Botox is the best treatment for this area. If the main problem is hanging, excess skin, the best treatment would be a facelift. And if the line is mostly due to fat accumulating outside the line, placing fat in the grooves would be a good treatment. Very often, these treatments are combined. If I'm going to do a facelift on someone with severe marionette's lines, I will usually recommend putting some fat in the lines at the same time. And if the person also has a very active, attached muscle in this area I will recommend Botox as well. Usually in younger patients, this line is primarily formed by muscular activity and Botox is my first choice of treatment. Once patients get into their late forties, however, usually at least some of the line is caused by hanging skin or fat that has slid down over the years due to gravity. In that case Botox may improve the line a tiny bit and a combination treatment is probably the best choice. Most serious problem areas in the face are best approached by a combination of procedures.

The forty-year-old patient in Figs. 69 through 74 illustrates the use of Botox in this area well. In Figs. 69 and 70 she is smiling her normal smile before and after injection. She did not like the extra little lines she was beginning to form running downward below the corners of her mouth. The good thing was these lines were just beginning to form. They weren't caused so much by hanging skin or fat pulled down by gravity but mostly by her muscles, which directly pulled down on her skin. You can see in her after photo that her smile has been cleaned up and the extra little lines are nearly gone. These lines were the beginnings of serious marionette's lines and this should help to prevent their formation. This patient was also a bit of a "chin talker" but did not have much of a cobblestone pattern, just a few dimples along the lower chin and a prominent wedge of muscle across her lower chin (Fig. 71). In Fig. 72 she can no longer make this expression. If you look back now at Figs. 69 and 70 you will notice that the shape of her chin has subtly changed. Since this wad of muscle across her lower chin no longer dominates her smile, her chin appears less wide and is more vertically oriented. The last two photos (Figs. 73 and 74) were taken after asking her to show me her lower teeth. This is a face most people make while brushing their lower teeth. The sharp indentations made by these downward pull-ing muscles are gone. This will help to prevent her from prematurely aging in this area.

But I don't inject only the muscle at the corners of the mouth to correct lines. Some people have a tendency when they smile to pull the corners of the mouth down. This is almost the opposite of the Mona Lisa smile. They're not trying to look unpleasant; it's just the way their muscles work. Most patients don't like this appearance. They look at photographs of themselves from a happy celebration and think, "I don't really look like that." But they do. This muscle at the corner that helps to create the marionette's lines is the primary muscle for pulling down the corners of the mouth. When this muscle is relaxed, the corners of the mouth turn up slightly both when resting and when smiling. This is something that most patients like. After smoothing the wrinkle lines, it is the leading benefit from this treatment. But some people get it just for the corners of the mouth. A model from Europe, who is a regular patient of mine, used to be shot in almost every photograph not smiling. That's because she's never liked her smile. She had a rather severe canine smile where she pulled her upper lip up very high above her teeth. At the same time, she also pulled down severely on the corners of her mouth. When she smiled, she actually looked as though she were in pain. So I injected the LAN muscle to lower her central upper lip and the muscle below the corners of her mouth to turn the corners of her mouth up. Now, she has a classic Mona Lisa smile. This is not one of the most common uses for Botox, but in the right patient it can produce a tremendous result.

There are other "smile problems" that Botox can work on. The woman in Figs. 65 through 68 did not like the extra dimpling in her cheeks and around the corners of her mouth when smiling with her mouth closed. They gave her a sort of smirking appearance. They were caused mostly by facial muscles that were directly attached to the un-dersurface of her skin, causing these extraneous ripples and dents when she smiled. As she was in her fifties, a little bit of sagging skin and loss of facial fat was also to blame, but not enough to make Botox ineffective.

Her closed-mouth smile shows the extra dents almost totally removed. She has a much cleaner, more youthful appearance around the mouth. The other important point is that when she smiles with her mouth open (Fig. 68) she has a completely normal, unaffected smile.

One of the most common complaints patients have when they walk into my office is the lip lines that develop radiating outward from their upper and lower lips. And while dermabrasion, laser resurfacing, and chemical peeling are options for these lines, the most common way to treat them is with an injection of a filler material like collagen. These lines, commonly called smokers' lines, are formed in two ways. Every time we purse our lips or sip from a straw (or smoke a cigarette), the muscle that runs in a circle around the mouth contracts. When it contracts, it bunches up the skin and forms these short lines. There is not a lot of fat between the muscle and skin in this area, so the crinkles in the muscle get transmitted to the surface of the skin. But something else creates the lines as well. As we age, our lips actually shrink. If you've stood in front of a mirror and thought to yourself that your lips used to be bigger, you were right. So the lines are formed both by the action of the muscle and the fact that the skin in this area forms an envelope around the lips. Since the contents of that envelope get smaller and smaller, the envelope wrinkles more easily.

There are two primary ways to attack this problem. One: stop the muscle from wrinkling the skin. Two: fill the envelope back up so that its surface is smooth. Not surprisingly, most patients want the envelope filled back up. This both makes the lines less noticeable and it also restores the volume of the lip. When it is done well, the results are excellent and very natural. Some patients balk when I suggest lip injections of collagen. Collagen looks bad in the lips when it is overdone. I reassure patients that the only time they notice it on others is when it is overdone. You've seen lots of lips with collagen but you just didn't realize it because it was done in a natural fashion.

So when do I inject Botox into the lips? If a patient wants a quick way to make the lines less obvious but does not want the lips to be any bigger at all, Botox is the best choice. Sometimes I will inject a patient's lips with collagen and the lines only get a little less obvious. Why did this happen? The depth and severity of the lines determine how much collagen might be needed. For instance, in an older patient with very wrinkled, shrunken lips, a lot of collagen might be required to get rid of the lines. Judgment is the key. These patients would be very upset if I squirted enough collagen into their lips to smooth them out as much as possible. They would look ridiculous. In these cases, a fair amount of collagen and a little Botox give the best no-downtime solution. The patient in Figs. 99 and 100 did not want to go through the skin testing that collagen requires to make sure that the patient is not allergic to it. If you are allergic to collagen, it is much better to have a small red, swollen lump in your forearm (where the skin test is placed) than a big, red, swollen face. Since we were injecting other areas of the face, she wanted to try this one too. In her after picture, she is not able to wrinkle her lips as she could beforehand. Although she was still making some lines (the after picture was taken two months after treatment), I did not give her a touch-up injection. In this area overinjecting could have disastrous consequences. Many of my patients who achieve good cosmetic results tell me the same thing—that they can speak and eat and drink from a straw just fine. But they have to concentrate a bit while performing these tasks because the lip feels weak to them. If they had had just a little more weakening, they would have real problems. This procedure is not for everybody.

A Smoother Neck

Even though you may not have heard about it—and many doctors don't realize it—Botox can produce gratifying results in the neck. I remember telling a plastic surgeon about seven years ago what great results I was having using Botox in the neck. He didn't believe it. He argued with me for several minutes, saying that only surgery could improve the aging neck.

To see why Botox works so well in the neck, it's necessary to know a little bit about the anatomy of the neck. The neck is covered by skin that is fairly thin relative to that of the face. This skin very loosely adheres to the structures underneath it so you can pinch it and pull it quite easily. In most people, underneath this skin is a thin layer of fat that can sometimes be quite concentrated; most is usually directly behind the chin. Below this fat is what I think is the key structure to aging in the neck: it is a flat, thin, smooth sheet of muscle that starts below the ears and acts as a sling to hold up the deeper structures of the neck. But this sling usually is not complete. The sling starts below the ears and progresses toward the middle of the neck but usually doesn't quite meet up with the muscle from the other side of the neck. So you have two separate sheets of muscle that end up an inch or two apart in the middle of the neck. The muscle fibers within these sheets are oriented vertically. These muscle fibers run from the chin straight back to the Adam's apple and then curve downward toward the floor.

The areas supported and covered and not so well supported or covered by the muscle are key. So is the muscle's orientation. These two important elements illustrate why Botox can work so well in the neck. This becomes obvious when you look at the profile of a youthful neck. In a youthful person who is not overweight, you see a clean jaw line and just below that jaw is fairly taut skin that goes back toward the neck almost parallel to the ground. Then this skin is bent at almost 90 degrees and covers the front surface of the neck going down over the Adam's apple until it reaches the collarbones. A youthful neck has a fairly sharp angle to it.

When I do a facelift, there are lots of different techniques to improve the neck. Very often, the area that is not supported by the muscle begins to sag a bit earlier than the portion of the neck that is supported: muscle is a lot stronger than skin when it comes to holding things up and resisting gravity. Through an incision just behind the chin, the edges of the muscle are often sutured together fairly tightly. This creates a fairly firm floor to support the structures in the neck above it. If there's a little extra fat concentrated behind the chin, that is removed at the same time so that the neck skin redrapes over this new taut muscular floor. This technique helps to re-create that sharp angle we were just talking about. But usually a little something is added to this technique. Usually, at the area toward the curve of the neck skin from horizontal to vertical, just past where the last stitch holding the muscle together is placed, the muscle is divided. Sometimes it's incised, or just weakened, but I usually prefer to actually remove a small section of this muscle.

You may wonder, if this muscle is so strong and helps to support whatever is beneath it, why would I want to deliberately weaken it. It goes back to the orientation of the muscle's fibers. If that section of muscle isn't removed, that muscle will continue to pull down on the neck, weakening the strong floor that I have just built. Even if you haven't had surgery, the downward pull of this muscle has a very negative effect on your neck. So there are three different aspects about this neck muscle that make it just right for Botox injection.

The two cords that most people begin to see going down the middle of their neck in their mid to late thirties are the edges of the muscle that we've been talking about. Sometimes these cords look like parallel strings attached behind the chin running down the neck. Initially, they are only visible when someone is straining or speaking loudly or forcefully. With time, these cords become present during any type of speech and then, finally, they are there all the time. Since that edge of the muscle toward the middle of the neck isn't attached to anything, it just hangs there. Over the years this muscle becomes thicker at its rolled-up edge. That thickening of the muscle pushing and pulling against the skin is the cord that you can see from the outside. Since these cords are made of muscle, they can be treated with Botox. When examining or injecting a patient, I'll ask her to show me her lower teeth. When she makes this face, this neck muscle contracts. Although primarily a job of the chin muscles, this neck muscle can also help to pull down the lower lip and corners of the mouth. I'll look at and feel the muscle on the neck as well as the skin. As long as the cords are primarily caused by the muscle, I will pinch that muscle between my fingers and, holding it in place, inject just the edges of that muscle with some Botox. This usually does not take a large amount of Botox, just enough to weaken the thickened edge of this muscle. If this muscle is overinjected with Botox, it can no longer hold up and support the structures of the neck. This can cause the neck to sag even farther. So while it's never good to overdo any area with Botox, a light dose is critical in the neck. An overinjected neck can give someone the appearance of a stork or a swallow with loose hanging flesh beneath the jaw.

This is assuming that the other structures, namely the skin and fat of the neck, are okay. If the skin of your neck has been stretched for years and is loose and hanging, all the Botox in the world isn't going to help you very much. It doesn't do anything to fat either. If you have a large collection of fat right under the chin, using Botox to weaken the muscle beneath it isn't going to do much. You may think that removing this fat will improve your result, and you'd be right most of the time. Clearly, if someone is walking around with a rather large lump of fat under the chin and that fat is removed with liposuction, the person will look better. But this often leads to a minor secondary problem. And it all depends on how much fat is actually left in the neck. If the liposuction in the neck is overdone, that layer of fat between the muscle and skin is practically gone. In that instance, it allows every ripple and pull of that muscle to be transmitted to the surface of the skin. This frequently makes neck cords even more apparent. While unsightly, that lump of fat behind the chin prevented the world from seeing your neck cords. It can also lead to the appearance of having multiple small strings running down from the chin under the skin. These are just different individual muscle fibers from the neck muscle that are now visible since its overlying layer of fat padding has been removed.

Now, let's say that too much fat hasn't been removed, that the liposuction was well done. Even so, some of the padding has been removed. So if someone had relatively heavy neck cords before the liposuction they probably would not have been seen. But after a well-done fat removal procedure, these heavy cords may now be visible. This is not an argument against liposuction. When well done, its results are outstanding. And in this hypothetical patient, they would still probably look better. But if the patient now has heavy cords where none were visible previously, the person may not be so thrilled with the result. This is where Botox comes in. Relaxing these two cords with a little Botox works very well in these post-liposuction patients. Now their lump of fat and their cords are gone.

Liposuction is not the only operation that works well with Botox injection of the neck cords. Face- and necklifts also work synergistically with Botox. Skin tightened previously with surgery, when the cords start to come back, is an excellent candidate for Botox. So there are two windows when Botox tends to have outstanding results in the neck. In the younger patient in her thirties to mid forties who does not have much extra skin the results are optimal. If this patient regularly relaxes these cords with Botox, it will also prevent the cords from stretching the overlying skin and thus may be useful for many additional years. This type of patient is seen in Figs. 79 and 80. She is shown straining before and after Botox injection to her neck cords. When this picture was taken, she was in her late thirties. She did not have any excess skin to mar her result. She is now in her mid-forties. Most women by this age have a bit of loose skin limiting their result. She does not. I believe that is mostly due to the fact that she has prevented her neck muscle from stretching out the overlying skin.

Figs. 81 and 82 show the neck of a woman in her late fifties before and after injection. She had a necklift by a different surgeon several years previously. Since she still did not have much excess skin at the time of this photo, she had an excellent result. I have been injecting this woman for six years. Not only has her excess neck skin not returned, but also the muscular floor just behind her skin is as taut as ever. Her weakened neck cords have neither stretched her skin nor pulled down the area just behind the chin. In this manner, Botox injections can extend the life of your facelift.

Since the muscle fibers in the neck run vertically, when the muscle contracts it contracts vertically. This can sometimes scrunch the skin, forming those faint horizontal lines that we begin to see in our neck in our thirties. Some of those lines exist primarily because of the muscle; some of those lines are formed every time we bend our head forward, moving the chin down toward the chest. When this happens, the skin creases. Since we make this motion a lot, especially while sleeping, we begin to develop permanent wrinkles across our neck. This is similar, although to a much lesser extent, to the wrinkles that we see in the palms of our hand. Every time we close our hand around something that skin folds and wrinkles. But these neck wrinkles are formed or at least made worse by the vertical scrunching action of the muscular sheet below the skin and fat of the neck. So, injecting a little bit of Botox above and below these lines helps to weaken the muscle a slight amount to make these horizontal lines less obvious. Again, care must be taken not to overinject the neck in this fashion for fear of weakening the muscular sling.

The shortest distance between two points is a straight line. Since the neck muscle starts at your chin and ends at your collarbone, that straight line would run directly between these two points. If this were the direction the skin of your neck took it would be unsightly. The entire contour of a youthful neck would be gone. So the muscle pulls and stretches your skin out of the angular configuration that is pleasing to the eye. This is another good reason to use Botox in the neck. It prevents your neck muscle from prematurely aging your neck. Since this muscle can also pull down on the chin and corners of the mouth, it also helps to prevent premature aging in these areas as well. But that doesn't mean you want all the muscle paralyzed, because some strength is needed in the muscle to support the neck. So I look for the areas that are pulling against the skin the hardest and trying to do the things that we don't want to have happen. Those are the areas that I target. But nothing is paralyzed here. I like to leave at least 90 percent of the muscle completely functional.

There's another advantage to using a great deal of care and very low doses of Botox in the neck. And that comes from some of the bad things you may have heard about Botox. It seems as if every newspaper magazine article I read that concerns Botox has to attempt to frighten the reader at least once. Usually, the neck stories are the most frightening of all. I have read stories about patients who had Botox in the neck and lost the ability to speak or swallow or hold their head up. I've never seen any of this. And it's hard for me to imagine that this could happen unless someone were injecting incredibly high doses of Botox indiscriminately into the neck. That wouldn't make sense for cosmetic purposes. There are also medical uses for Botox in the neck, such as for cervical dystonia or torticollis. These conditions involve spasms and contractions of larger, deeper muscles in the neck requiring deep, high doses. In these patients, complications certainly would be understandable. As far as difficulty swallowing goes, one of the best uses for Botox is for a condition called achalasia in which Botox is injected into the food pipe to *improve* swallowing.

4

THE GUIDE FOR GUYS

~~~~~~~~~~~~~~~~~~~~~~
~~~~~~~~~~~~~~~~~~~~~~

From news reports, magazine articles, and commercials you may have seen, you may have assumed that Botox was just for women. That's understandable. The reason that so much of the Botox media frenzy seems to be aimed at women is because they have more facelifts, liposuction, chemical peels, and collagen than men, so the advertising and information people have targeted them. It's just part of our culture. Don't expect to see too many men's magazines with cover stories about Botox. It just wouldn't fly. Despite a growing trend of shirtless male models with rippled abs on their covers, you won't see men's magazines featuring Botox. Why? Because men have fitness and health magazines while women have beauty magazines. What's inside? In both, it's about trying to be more attractive to members of the opposite sex, with accompanying conspiratorial guy talk or girl talk. But there's no such thing as a men's beauty magazine.

Men don't need to feel left out. If you've got a furrowed brow, a forehead that recalls Alfred E. Neuman, Clint Eastwood–style crow's feet, a chin that looks as if you fell asleep on a waffle iron, or what looks like two steel cables hanging from your lower chin trying to pull your neck down to the floor, Botox may work for you too. But just as a higher percentage of men go for certain plastic surgery operations like nose jobs and eye tucks, certain areas for Botox use are more popular with men.

The biggest reason for the difference in results between men and women when using Botox is the skin. Male skin is much thicker and heavier in the face than female skin. Then there's the skin that contains the beard, which is thicker and heavier still. This thick skin is less supple and responsive to the muscles beneath it. So it's a plus/minus situation. Over many years of muscles pulling on its undersurface, thicker skin does a better job resisting these forces. It also resists the fine lines and wrinkles much better than thinner skin. That's the good part. The not-so-great part is that when these forces are removed, you don't see as big a change since the forces didn't have that much influence on the skin in the first place. The thicker skin tends to hide what's going on underneath it. If you had a chainsaw on a table and covered it with a thin piece of silk, anyone would be able to tell what it was. But if that same chainsaw were covered with a heavy, thick piece of leather, only the Amazing Kreskin or for the younger reader, Miss Cleo, would have any idea what lay beneath it.

The other downside of this thick skin is the effect gravity has on it. The heavier, thicker skin in a man's lower face tends to get pulled down more strongly than the thinner, beardless skin of his upper face. That's why frequently you'll see a man in his sixties or seventies who looks pretty good across the upper two-thirds of his face but has shar-pei smile lines, hound-dog jowls, and a quivering, flopping turkey neck. This heavy skin in the lower face tends to limit the effectiveness of Botox in these areas for men.

As far as the smile lines go, in general, I think this is the least effective area on a man's face for Botox for a couple of reasons. One, most men start to get smile lines in their early thirties. The smile lines tend to be a bit heavier and thicker than those in women. A lot of this has to do with a heavy bearded skin being pulled down over the top of the smile lines by gravity. So, in a man, the smile lines tend to be caused more by heavy excess skin than the muscles that pull on and create the smile lines in the first place. Weakening the LAN muscle wouldn't help this very much and would just drop down a man's upper lip. Since men in general tend to have slightly smaller smiles and show less upper teeth than women, this would look really bad. You could go from showing the bottom third of your teeth to looking as if you'd forgotten to put your dentures in that day. And your smile lines wouldn't be any better.

Two, for whatever reason, smile lines are a little more accepted on men. It makes them look weathered, and rugged, which is considered attractive. If a woman at forty had no smile lines, people would say that she looked great. If a forty-year-old man didn't have any smile lines he would look quite odd. Not to say I haven't injected male smile lines with Botox. There's a small window, when the smile lines are just beginning to form and the heavy skin hasn't yet slid over the line creating an overhang, where Botox can be effective. But once smile lines become ingrained in a man's skin, I don't recommend Botox.

This is mirrored when it comes to injecting fillers in the smile lines for men. And the percentage of men who have collagen or other off-the-shelf fillers injected into their smile lines is fairly small. That's because, once these lines become fairly heavy, the fillers don't really do too much. My best results when injecting smile lines in men is with fat. It's a bit heavier, thicker, and longer lasting. The only drawback is the ten days to two weeks that you've got to hide from the neighbors. Unless you're known for getting into fights, it's hard to explain away the swelling below your nose and across your upper lip.

The neck also contains this heavy pulled-down skin. But I find my results in the neck are better than my results in the smile lines. Although you rarely go from the strong paired cord appearance to completely smooth as you do in women, the results are still pretty good. As long as the skin hasn't been permanently stretched out by the two cords of muscles running beneath it, you can still get a nice result. The obvious bonus, of course, is that when you weaken these two muscular cords you stop them from continually pulling down on the skin beneath the neck. This way you prevent your neck muscles from assisting gravity in its quest to give you a turkey neck. I find this works really well for men in their late thirties through their forties; it works especially well just below the chin. It is during our forties that most men start to develop a little jowling.

One of the things that is associated with a more youthful appearance in both sexes is having a clean jawline. That starts to go in our forties. The jawline starts with the chin; then right around and below each side of the chin the jawline is obscured for a few inches and then hopefully it reappears again farther back below your ear. That little bit of tissue that slides over your jawline obscuring it, is what people refer to as jowls. Jowls are a combination of things. Most people think that the jowls are mostly formed by skin that has slid over the jawline. That's not true. It's actually the heavier tissues below the skin like the fat and muscle that have slid over the jawline and pulled the skin along for the ride. That's why the best treatment for this area, in both sexes, is some variation of facelift surgery in which the deeper tissues of the fat and muscles are elevated to their previous homes in the cheek. If you noticed that it seems as though your cheekbones are not as big as they were twenty years ago, you are not seeing things. While it is unlikely that the size of your bones has changed, what has happened is the thick fat that used to sit on top of your cheekbones has slid down into your cheeks. The fat that used to be in your cheeks has slid down over the jaw and now rests peacefully in your jowls.

So what causes these heavy tissues to slide over the edge of the cliff and dangle? Mostly gravity. But I think in men more than women, the upper muscles of the neck contribute to this decline to a greater extent. These muscles actually help to pull the fat and muscles from above over the jawline. In some patients, these muscles can even help to pull the corners of the mouth down a small amount. So injecting these muscles can actually help stave off the early turkey neck and jowls until you are solidly middle-aged.

Since wrinkling and dimpling in the chin are more directly caused by chin muscles rather than gravity or heavy skin, they respond well to Botox, even in men's thick skin. The thicker male skin doesn't transmit the wrinkling of the muscle beneath it to the surface very well, so men tend to have this problem less frequently than women. But when it's there, it responds really well.

There are also many differences that one needs to keep in mind when injecting the upper face in men as compared to women. Just as the frowning muscles are the keystone to a good Botox injection in women, the same is true in men. Just as in women, the muscles of the brow pull the brows together and down. But as opposed to causing fine wrinkles, in men that fine wrinkle is resisted by the thick skin. But what will happen after years of pulling is that a deep furrrow seems to develop almost overnight. All that pulling during all those years has finally deeply indented the skin. Botox works really well for this problem. However, once this deep furrow is established, it usually doesn't go completely away with just Botox. Sometimes younger men who may have thinner skin can get total clearance of the lines. In the vast majority of cases, the furrow is improved enough that the patient doesn't want a secondary procedure other than repeated Botox injections. But to really get a smooth appearance in this area, it often takes a secondary treatment such as collagen or fat injections to plump up this deeper, more estab-lished groove.

When this is done, I get a lot of feedback from my male patients that may surprise you. Women are usually just happy that they look so much better. They are happy that they don't see that wrinkle or crease between their eyes anymore. Men often say something like "People aren't afraid of me anymore." Another common remark is that things seem to be going much better for them in the workplace. This is especially true for men who are at all involved in sales, which is the process of selling themselves. Depending on the physiognomy of the face, furrows between the eyes can convey concerned concentration, attentiveness, anger, or rage. These last two are obviously not ideal for anyone involved in a people business. I've had salesmen tell me that their income has gone up 50 percent since they started using Botox, although I think this may be due more to the effect on their psyche and self-image than on their face. I have also had men tell me that they can't go to work without it.

This was the case with the man in Figs. 5 through 8. In Figs. 5 and 6 he is frowning before and after Botox injections to his frowning muscles only. This is a standard result for this type of injection. But the real change is seen in Figs. 7 and 8. He is seen at rest in these photos. By just weakening his brow there has been a total change in his demeanor. He no longer appears to be glowering but it almost seems as though there is a hint of a smile in his picture after treatment. But he is not smiling. The entire result is due to eliminating that resting tension in his frowning muscles.

For whatever reason, there is still a little more stigma attached to a man who does something medical or surgical about his looks than to a woman. Because of this, even men who just want to look better will often blame their wives, girlfriends, or jobs for the final push that got them into my office. I can't tell you how many of my consultations have started out with my asking a male patient what we're going to talk about that day. So often, the first words out of their mouths are "My wife doesn't like this turkey neck," or "My girlfriend thinks the bump in my nose is too big," or "There are some younger new hotshots at work and I just can't afford to seem old around them." Very often what they say is true. But a lot of men have a hard time just admitting that they want to look better. Getting a man to admit he just wants to look better is about as easy as getting one to ask for directions.

Besides the frowning area, another terrific area for Botox injection in men is the forehead. Men often develop heavy horizontal lines across the forehead much earlier in their lives than women. There is a reason for this. Typically, our eyebrows sit a lot lower across the bones that make up the top of the eye socket than women's brows. Our brows are also flatter and less curved. Sometimes these heavy flat brows crowd our upper eyelids. We don't even realize that it bothers our eyelids. But it does. The muscles in our eyelids that open our eyes are very delicate and thin wisps of muscle. This muscle doesn't like trying to hold up the heavy skin of our brows. So our brows push down on our eyelids until our eyelids send a signal back to our brain that they've had enough. The signal then comes back to your forehead muscles to pull up on your

eyebrows, giving your eyelids much needed relief. So the eyebrow weight
is off the eyelids for a few moments until gravity starts to pull it down,
down, down back on top of the lids again. Then the process starts all
over. Pulling your eyebrows up forcefully a few thousand times a day
with your forehead muscles tends to put some pretty good creases in
your forehead at an early age.

Weakening the forehead muscles will obviously help with these lines.
The forehead muscles won't be able to beat up your skin and the constant resting tone in the forehead will be less, allowing the skin to stretch
back out. But this does not come without a cost. If your forehead muscles
are not pulling up so well on your eyebrows anymore, they'll tend to sit
even lower on your face and bother your eyelids even more. That's why
I will never completely inject the forehead muscles in a man. You have
to understand that there is no free lunch. Overweakening of these muscles will push the brows down even lower and flatter and hold them
right on top of the eyelids. Not only will your eyelids revolt, but this is
not an attractive appearance. So what can you do? Well, the first thing
is to be very selective about the areas on the forehead to weaken. When
someone looks at you, the gaze is usually focused down the center of
your face. People tend to notice forehead wrinkles in the middle of the
forehead more than forehead wrinkles on the outside portions of the
forehead. Because of this, I usually weaken the forehead muscles in men
directly over the nose. This helps with the deepest and most obvious of
the forehead lines. It also doesn't weaken the portions of the muscles
directly over the eyebrows. Those portions are still working. But if you
just weaken the middle part of the forehead, something unusual happens. The rest of the forehead musculature realizes that part of it has
been weakened. Therefore, it tends to pull up even harder where it
hasn't been weakened. Injecting the forehead only right down the middle
can lead to the Mr. Spock, or when less severe, Jack Nicholson, look.
And in case you haven't noticed, Vulcans are not considered very attractive by earth women. And although Mr. Nicholson has a rakish, ras-
cally charm and is attractive to earth women, you are not Jack Nicholson.
You do not have any Academy Awards. You do not make twenty million

dollars per movie. You were not in *Easy Rider*. You are not that charming. Repeat, you are not Jack Nicholson.

If I notice that the outer forehead muscles are also quite strong, they get a little Botox as well. Not so much that the muscles won't pull at all and that the brows will sag. But just enough so that the outer brows don't try to fly away. The other important point to keep in mind when weakening a man's forehead is the group of muscles that pulls in the other direction, helping gravity to bring the eyebrows down. If you're going to weaken the muscles that are raising the eyebrows, you'd better be weakening the muscles pulling the eyebrows down. This way, I hope in the man with a severely wrinkled forehead to at least leave the eyebrows where they were when I started. For heavy wrinkles, the forehead has to be moderately weakened. This would surely result in drooping of the brows if every piece of muscle pulling down on the eyebrows were not weakened too. Usually, a man with forehead lines also has frown lines, so he wants that area injected too. But sometimes not. And occasionally I spend fifteen or twenty minutes trying to convince someone that he should let me inject his frowning muscles even though he doesn't have frown lines. I can't tell you have many times I've had a man come into my office and say that Botox was "no good" for him in the forehead. When I ask why, he invariably says it pushes his eyebrows way down and makes his eyes really tired at the end of the day. When I ask him if any other areas were injected, he says no. I usually will get him to let me try it my way. I've never had anyone come back and say he was sorry he let me try it.

The crow's feet area also works really well for men. Typically, men tend to have a full-fan-shaped crow's feet pattern. In other words, we wrinkle our skin from above the corner of the eye in the eyebrow around the corner of the eye down to the lower lid and upper cheek. This area responds really well to Botox as long as the lines are not heavily ingrained. Even when the lines are ingrained and a man has that sun-and-weather-beaten leathery appearance, these lines can at least be diminished by Botox. There are two things to be careful of here. If the upper part of the crow's feet is heavily injected, this can cause our old

friend Mr. Spock to come visiting again. That's because that upper portion of the crow's-feet muscle pulls down on the eyebrow. Weakening it
allows the eyebrow to pop up over the outer part of the eye. If I'm going
to weaken this area for crow's feet, I always weaken the outer part of
the forehead directly above it to prevent the forehead muscle from pulling up too much on the eyebrow. Another tricky area is at the other end
of the crow's feet fan. It's completely my opinion, but I think most men
look better with a little crow's feet coming down on their cheek. Older
men with no lines look a bit strange. Even when he was in his thirties,
Clint Eastwood had incredibly heavy crow's feet lines. Where would he
be without these lines or the ability to squint? If you overweaken this
lower part of the crow's feet, it may also make your smile seem a little
strange. Not because the Botox has seeped or drifted down into your
smiling muscles per se. But the bottom portion of the crow's feet muscle
also helps to pull up a tiny bit on the upper cheek. With all this, when
smiling, the face can have a sort of flat, droopy look. Not good.

The man in Figs. 51 through 54 had his frowning, forehead, and
crow's feet muscles injected. He is sixty-five years old. The first two
photos show the result that you can get in the frowning area even when
the wrinkles have been established for many years. They are improved
but not gone. If this gentleman wanted further smoothing of the area, a
little collagen would be my first choice. Figs. 13 C and D show his right
crow's feet area while smiling. Clearly, there is a nice improvement but
I did not try to get him completely smooth. A man like him would look
bizarre if he did not have any lines in this area. I especially like to leave
a few extra lines across the upper cheek. One, it looks good and two, it
allows him to fully lift up his cheek when he smiles. If you'll notice, I
injected his upper crow's feet more strongly than his lower. That was so
I could eliminate the hooding effect across his upper, outer eyelid. Now
when he smiles, his eyes stay open and aren't pinched closed beneath
the outer eyebrow.

Sometimes, the crow's feet are injected not because of the crow's feet
area per se but because of the forehead. If a man has severe wrinkling
of the forehead toward its outer portions and that is what is bothering

him, I change my pattern of injection. I will primarily inject the outer portion of the forehead. Then to prevent the middle part of the brows from being elevated into a quizzical appearance, the middle part of the forehead is also injected lightly. But if that's all that is done, the brows will really be pushed down on the outside of the eyes, giving you a little bit of the old Sylvester Stallone look. And once again, while it may work for Rocky or Rambo, it probably won't work for you. I inject a fair amount of Botox into the upper crow's feet area to prevent that muscle from pulling the outer eyebrow down. This way, the eyebrows stay where they started and the forehead wrinkles are improved.

Sometimes, I inject these three areas in men not because of lines at all. As I said before, men naturally have low flat brows. Some men have brows lower than others. Some men age more quickly than others, so their brows are really pulled down at a relatively early age. There is an operation that corrects this quite well. It's called a brow or forehead lift. There are a few different ways to do this operation but it usually involves putting at least some scars in the scalp just behind where a full hairline would be. The problem is by the time they're fifty, about 60 percent of men have had hair loss in this area. Even those who haven't had it may develop it in the years to come. For this reason, it is very unusual to do a browlift on a man. Occasionally, a man with a full head of hair and a good family history is unconcerned about the scars and will have the operation. Sometimes, a man who has had hair transplants will have the operation, since these hairs are not going anywhere. But most men don't fit into these categories. For this reason, they try to raise their brows without having surgery. The best way to do this is with Botox.

Figs. 47 through 50 show your author in his thirties after injections to his brow, forehead, and crow's feet area. Figs. 47 and 48 show me frowning before and after injection. As you can see, I prefer to inject myself very lightly (Hollywood style) so that I still have some motion. But I left myself with motion pulling my brows toward each other but not so much motion pulling them down. I can still make the two faint vertical frown lines but not the horizontal one at the bridge of my nose. I also weakened my forehead slightly and only the upper portion of my crow's feet. For now, I like my crow's feet. They are there when I smile and not apparent in repose. Figs. 49 and 50 show the real effect of my injections. At rest, as you can see in Fig. 49, I don't have much in the way of wrinkles but my brows are a bit low and crowding my eyelids. Where before my brows obscured the edges of my eyelids, after injection you can see my eyelids all the way across my eyes. Granted, this is a minimal elevation of my brows, but that is all I wanted. Anything more than this would have been overdone and a little feminine. Besides not raising the brows too much, care was taken not to increase the slight arch that I already had.

This works pretty much the same way it does in women. The idea is to weaken or sometimes even completely paralyze all of the muscle segments that are pulling down on the eyebrows. There are thirteen different segments of muscle that do this. This requires a pretty thorough knowledge of anatomy on the part of the doctor, but that's not all it requires. The anatomy in these areas varies widely from patient to patient. Very rarely during an operation do you see all the muscles exactly as they were drawn in an anatomy textbook. So you have to do a little detective work and educated guesswork. I will have the patient make many different odd facial expressions. I will ask him to repeat these expressions over and over for a few minutes, telling him to relax his face in between the grimaces, frowns, and smiles. What I am trying to do is visualize where these muscle segments are and which muscle segments are stronger than others. That way I can make an educated guess, based on years of injecting Botox and years of looking at these muscles during surgery, as to where my needle should go with how much Botox. While you would think that the maximal elevation one could achieve would occur if you left the forehead muscles completely uninjected and at full strength, you would be wrong. If you inject part of this musculature, the other parts tend to pull more strongly. So I will weaken the forehead that is not directly responsible for pulling up on the brows to get the areas above the brows to pull more strongly. But you cannot have just the portion directly over the brows pulling more strongly. That would arch and feminize the brow, not a good look. You want the entire forehead area over the brow pulling at the same strength, trying to keep the brows straight. In this way, I can usually raise the brow a few millimeters in men. I can't raise the brow the full six millimeters that I can in women. I think the reason is that the brow is just so much heavier in men and that it even feels a little more densely attached to the bone beneath it. So the results are not quite as startling. But in a way that's a good thing. No one of either sex looks good with an overly raised brow up in the middle of his or her forehead. But certainly women can get away with a high brow a lot better than men can. I think the worst, most striking bad result of surgery on men is the overdone browlift (followed closely by the overdone needle-nose rhinoplasty and wind tunnel face-lift). Not being able to raise the male brow too severely is probably a good thing.

Speaking about overly raised brows, I lied to you a little bit earlier. I said that I never completely inject the forehead, totally weakening its muscles. That's not exactly true. In a normal patient, I would never do that. But some patients have been referred to me who've had poor out-comes from surgery done elsewhere. Sometimes I do completely paralyze the forehead after a browlift that was too severe. I know I'm repeating myself, but if you take one thing away from this book I think that this should be it. *Nothing looks good when it's overdone.* Overdone facelifts, overdone browlifts, overdone collagen resulting in gigantic lips, and over-done Botox should not have a place in normal society. So occasionally I am referred someone whose brows have been artificially raised too high. In that person, I will completely paralyze the forehead. Usually, I can drop the brows a few millimeters in this way as long as I leave all the muscles pulling down on the brows at full strength. And then, hope-fully, the patient can avoid the "somebody just poured ice water down my back" look.

5

SELECTING A PRACTITIONER

Plastic Surgeon, Dermatologist, Ophthalmologist, or Nurse?

You've decided to take the plunge and schedule your consultation for Botox injections. Whom do you call? Well, as a plastic surgeon, you may expect me to be biased. I've tried to avoid that bias in this book. In fact, I think that it is surgical bias that pushes some plastic surgeons to tell patients that Botox isn't really good for the neck and lower face, and that they need a face- or necklift. I think this happened for a while with the upper face as well. But the tremendous results with Botox over so many years in so many patients have rendered that point moot. I've tried to avoid any anti-dermatologist, pro–plastic surgeon bias in this book. In fact, I'm often asked to recommend a Botox injector when I'm unable to fit someone into my schedule, and I think I recommend plastic surgeons and dermatologists equally often.

I have attended meetings with both plastic surgeons and dermatologists. I'm familiar with some of the sniping that goes on in regard to each other's specialties. Dermatologists will often complain that plastic surgeons inject Botox poorly. They say that this is due to the fact that to plastic surgeons anything short of a full facelift, necklift, and eyelid surgery procedure is seen as not really plastic surgery and not worth their time. That having to run into a room with a little needle and squirt in a few drops of liquid is an inconvenience, a pain in the neck, something to be tolerated and done as quickly as possible. The conventional wisdom is that plastic surgeons cannot be bothered with such an insignificant little injection. Because many plastic surgeons do not make Botox a focus of their practice, they rush through it as quickly as possible. I do not do that in my own practice, and colleagues I know well and respect do not do it in theirs. However, like a lot of clichés, they become clichés because they're partly true. I would be dishonest if I said that there was not a shred of truth to these statements. I'm sure that the occasional plastic surgeon who is always trying to keep up with a variety of new surgical techniques probably doesn't pay much attention to what is going on with Botox injections. And I'm sure that some plastic surgeons occasionally only inject Botox because they see it as a necessary evil to keep their patients happy. Fortunately, I think these plastic surgeons are few and far between.

Plastic surgeons who do a fair amount of Botox frequently have a bias against their dermatologist colleagues. Their most common complaint is that dermatologists don't inject Botox well because they don't know the anatomy of the muscles that they are trying to inject. I'm sure this is not true for the majority of dermatologists. Surgeons say that even if dermatologists studied the anatomy at length from a textbook, the anatomy is always a little bit different in the actual patient. Dermatologists do not see these muscles on a regular basis as plastic surgeons do. Even if the dermatologist were go into an anatomy lab and dissect these muscles on a cadaver, the experience would not be the same because these muscles are always a little different in the living patient. What helped me a great deal in 1991, when I was just beginning to inject Botox, was the fact that I literally saw the muscles that I wanted to hit with my Botox needle on a daily basis. I think this probably gives the plastic surgeon a slight advantage over the dermatologist for the initial several injections. I believe the learning curve for plastic surgeons isn't as steep as it is for dermatologists. But I have absolutely no doubt that with careful observation and a little experience, any conscientious dermatologist can become a proficient injector of Botox. I'm frequently asked by my regular patients in New York who may be traveling for extended periods or by my out-of-town patients who are unable to travel to New York to see me for a particular injection, to recommend a Botox injector in another city. I have a relatively short list of doctors that I feel comfortable sending my patients to but it is split about fifty-fifty between plastic surgeons and dermatologists.

A trend that has been accelerating over the past few years is one for the worse, in my opinion. It's something that has been covered by the *New York Times* and *60 Minutes*. The trend is for other physicians to move into the plastic surgery arena. This is happening for several reasons: one is the decreased reimbursement from HMOs and the increased overhead expense of fighting with them and filing multiple reports and bills. Ask any doctors who are forced to deal with them on a regular basis and they will tell you that managed care has managed to dramatically increase the bureaucracy and red tape of medicine. Steadily rising malpractice premiums, due to ever-increasing awards given at malpractice cases, have raised their overhead even higher. On a patient-by-patient basis over the last ten years, these physicians have much less money coming in and much more going out and are working longer hours. In order to make up for the shortfall, many have turned to plastic surgery.

It's not hard to figure out why. Money. A premium can be charged for plastic surgery procedures. Throw in the fact that it's paid for up front by the patient, and that the doctor doesn't need to hire an army of people to file reports and fight with insurance companies, and it's a no-brainer. If doctors want to change the focus of their practice of medicine in midcareer to plastic surgery, I support that wholeheartedly. As long as they apply for, are accepted by, and complete a certified plastic surgery residency program. After all, if you want to call yourself a plastic surgeon, shouldn't you complete a plastic surgery residency? Would you want the ophthalmologist doing your cataract surgery to be someone who did not complete one day of an ophthalmology residency? Would you want the radiologist reading your mammograms to have done a radiology residency? Would you care if the neurosurgeon trying to remove a brain tumor from your mother completed an approved residency in neurological surgery? Unfortunately, that is a very rare occurrence for the newly minted "plastic surgeon." More likely, this physician has attended a weekend course or watched videotapes of plastic surgery procedures. My total training period for plastic surgery was eight years after medical school. It is only my opinion, but I do not think that you can achieve the level of knowledge, judgment, and proficiency required to safely perform plastic surgery by simply attending courses. In prior chapters, I talked about the muscular anatomy of the face and neck. Besides the strictly anatomical viewpoint, it is also important to realize the different relative strengths and contributions of these many muscles to facial expressions and lines. This comes about from years of studying faces, and is something that both plastic surgeons and dermatologists have done.

Another group of physicians that I would recommend are specially trained ophthalmologists. I first heard about Botox from an ophthalmologist—one of the Carruthers is an ophthalmologist—and other doctors that I know have been injecting it for least ten years also were often ophthalmologists. That's because, when it first came on the market, Botox was primarily an ophthalmologic drug. Some ophthalmologists undergo an additional year of specialty training involving plastic surgery around the eye. They are referred to as oculoplastic surgeons. This group of ophthalmologists I would also recommend without hesitation for Botox injections around the eye area.

Another rather new development in Botox injections is the fact that nurses are doing more and more of them. On this issue, I'm sort of split down the middle. In other words, I think a talented nurse under the close supervision of an expert physician injector can become, in time, a proficient Botox injector. But I would not recommend seeing a nurse on her own who is performing injections without supervision, guidance, and follow-up closely directed by a physician.

Beware of "Bogus Boards" and Bargain Botox

When patients discuss a physician's credentials, they often say that their physicians are "board-certified." But if you ask these patients what this really means, they're often unsure. They seem to think there is one large board that certifies physicians of different specialties. They are partially right. Obviously, the training and board examinations that a dermatologist (a subspecialty of internal medicine) and a plastic surgeon (a subspecialty of surgery) undergo are quite different. There are separate boards to certify physicians in each specialty. But there is one main board that has all these other smaller boards under its umbrella—the American Board of Medical Specialties. This board determines which other boards can become member boards. In other words it determines the need and qualifications of boards to be recognized. This is an important distinction. Without this distinction there would be no way to tell which of the hundreds of "boards" are recognized boards and which boards are not. Here is a list of the twenty-four recognized boards at this time: allergy and immunology, anesthesiology, colon and rectal surgery, dermatology, emergency medicine, family practice, internal medicine, medical genetics, neurological surgery, nuclear medicine, obstetrics and gynecology, ophthalmology, orthopedic surgery, otolaryngology, pathology, pediatrics, physical medicine and rehabilitation, plastic surgery, preventive medicine, psychiatry, radiology, surgery, thoracic surgery, and urology. Any other board, even if its name differs only slightly from one of the previous twenty-four boards, is not a recognized board. You can call 1-866-ASK-ABMS for information regarding physicians belonging to one of the member boards of the American Board of Medical Specialties. They also have an excellent Web site at ABMS.org. Whereas there are 24 recognized boards, there are over 180 unrecognized boards and that number is climbing.

Dermatology and plastic surgery are two of the boards recognized by the American Board of Medical Specialties. If a patient were to ask me for a referral, I would recommend that he or she see a physician certified by one of these two boards or a specially trained ophthalmologist. While unrecognized boards certainly have excellent physicians (some of whom I have recommended to my patients) it would be difficult for me to recommend them as a group.

One of the reasons for the proliferation of unrecognized or "bogus" boards, as they are sometimes called, is the ease with which they can sometimes be created. If you hire an attorney and have a few extra dollars, you can form a corporation. Anyone who forms a corporation can name that corporation basically whatever he wants so long as that name has not already been taken. That person can then claim to be a "board." For instance, tomorrow some physician could incorporate himself. Typically, an incorporated physician names the corporation his name, M.D., P.C. But he doesn't have to. He could name his corporation the "American Board of Botulinum Toxin Injectors." He would then appoint himself president of that board. He could then invite other physicians to fill out a few forms, state in writing that they've done a few Botox injections, pay him $1,000, and he would then send them a large certificate proclaiming that they are board-certified. Frequently, these boards have a name only slightly different from the name of a recognized board. Maybe that's what they wanted to name their board all along. Maybe they want to give the impression that their members are incredibly specialized. Maybe they are just trying to confuse you. But I don't want to give you a wholly negative impression. Some unrecognized boards do seek to apply objective standards and have good physicians as members. However, I could not in good conscience recommend that a patient find an injector by primarily seeking a member of an unrecognized board.

I've seen many ads for bargain Botox. I've seen many ads, in fact, for $99 Botox. At the time that this book went to print, a vial of Botox was sold to the physician for $392. Depending on how many areas of a patient are injected and how much is injected into each area, sometimes the patient receives close to an entire vial. There's only one manufacturer and distributor of Botox in the United States and the per-vial price is never discounted, not even for physicians who, like myself, use extremely high volumes of Botox. So how can someone be doing Botox injections for $99? The answer is simple. Since Botox, when it is delivered, is merely a small amount of powder in the bottom of the vial, it needs to be reconstituted. That is, a small amount of saltwater needs to be added to the powder to turn it into a solution that can be injected with a syringe. It is up to the physician how much saltwater is used. Some physicians like to argue that only their amount or their dilution per vial is the proper way to inject. I disagree with that. I think there's plenty of room for personal taste in this area. What is important is the total dose of the active ingredient that is injected. Patients who have been injected by other physicians before they have come to me often say that the doctor needed one or one half of a syringe for this or that area. That information doesn't mean anything without knowing how much that doctor likes to dilute his Botox. Clearly, with an ultra-low-cost Botox deal, you can't be getting the right amount of the drug for such a small price. I've seen several patients in my practice who went to a bargain Botox injector. Invariably they tell me that nothing happened or very little happened. Some patients were embarrassed for visiting that clinic in the first place and just let it go at that. Others returned to the clinic. These patients are usually told the same story: that they must be immune to Botox. I will then ask these patients to let me reinject them. And I've never had one that did not respond. During my eleven years of injecting patients, I've never injected one person I know of who was immune to Botox.

Another trend that has been springing up is the Botox party. This idea actually sprang from the mind of one public relations agent who had a client who was a young dermatologist and who needed a novel way of promoting himself. Well, it worked.

While not up to the sterile standards of an operating room, an office examination or treatment room still has a few standards to meet. Though not sterile, it is considered a clean room. There are regulations about this. There can't be any carpets (too difficult to disinfect) and there must be a sink for the physician to wash his hands. My rooms are cleaned by a professional cleaning service to keep bacteria to a minimum. This is not the same kind of atmosphere that you find in a hair salon or friend's home or gym. That's right, some Botox parties are now being held in gyms. One of the few things I prohibit my patients from doing after an injection is raising their heart rate, so getting Botox in the middle of your workout is not a good idea.

But say the Botox party is being held at the doctor's office. I would still be a bit wary. You read about people being served champagne and cosmopolitans while they wait for their turn in the doctor's chair. One of the things I try to provide for my patients is a relaxed environment. Sure, it's good for their psyche and their overall experience in my office but there is another, more important reason. When you're anxious, your heart races and the blood flows a little more forcefully through the tissues that I'm injecting. I don't want that. In fact, I want the opposite. I want the circulation to be at a minimum in the areas that I place my Botox. For two good reasons. One, with an increase in the circulation the risk of bruising is much greater. These little muscles have a tremendous blood supply compared to the fat and skin around them. I always ice my patients along their areas to be injected before touching them with a needle. Most of my patients are thankful for this, thinking the main reason I do it is their comfort. Yes, it does help with the discomfort of the needle going through the skin. But the main reason I do it is to cut down on their risk of bruising. Before I started icing patients, about 10 percent of my patients were bruised after injection. After I began conscientiously icing down everyone before injection, that rate fell to 4 percent. That's because the coldness of the ice induces the blood vessels to shrivel up. This makes it less likely that a needle will touch one of the blood vessels and cause a bruise. The second and even more important reason to me is the overall temporary decrease in circulation of the area. When I inject someone with Botox, I am very precise about where I place it. Not only into which muscles, but into which parts of which muscles. So I want it to stay where I put it. There's a greater chance for this if the circulation in that area is at a minimum.

So the excitement and activity and chatter immediately before flopping into your doctor's chair is not good. But what's far worse is the alcohol. Alcohol dilates your superficial blood vessels. This tremendously increases the circulation to your skin and superficial tissues. That is why a drink on a cold night will warm you up: it dilates the blood vessels to the skin, bringing warm blood flooding through these areas. Increasing your blood flow through the muscles with excitement and alcohol before a Botox injection is a bad idea.

Lastly, think about the physician himself. If this physician were such a good Botox injector, what is he doing hanging around in the evening to try to scrape up a few more patients? When I finish my day, usually around 6 or 6:30 P.M., I do not want to do any more Botox injections. I've been injecting people all day long. I don't feel like staying after hours, setting up a bar, and ordering in sushi just so I can inject a few more patients. In fact, my room for new patients is already very limited. So you should think hard about whom you really want behind the needle when you get Botox injections.

The "Botox day" is a little different from the Botox party. During a Botox day, the physician tries to group together Botox patients so that there is no Botox wasted (it has a short shelf life). That is good—for your doctor. And while scheduling your appointments around these days at least is a sign your doctor has other Botox patients to schedule you with, doctors who do a lot of Botox do not have Botox days. That is because every day is Botox day.

Do Your Homework

So now you've decided to go ahead and schedule your consultation for Botox. Whom do you call? I think that the best way to find a good Botox injector is to ask your friends or a doctor you trust. With the fading stigma attached to plastic surgery and especially to something as quick and efficient as Botox injections, many people do not keep their use of it a secret. People you trust, and have been injected, and who look good to you, I think, are your best source for unbiased information. I would warn you to be careful taking recommendations from hairdressers, facialists, manicurists, and so forth, as frequently they may have a financial interest in referring you to a specific doctor. Even if they don't have a direct fee-for-service type of financial arrangement, these people often receive free treatments by physicians in exchange for referring patients. Another poor way to find a physician is through an advertisement. If that physician is such a good Botox injector and injects so many people, why does that physician need to advertise? I think one of the worst reasons to go to a doctor is because you read about that doctor in a magazine article or newspaper or saw him on a quick segment on the news. As I've been on the lecture circuit for a few years teaching Botox, I've met and served on the same panels with just about every other person that I would consider to be an expert in this field. These physicians are at the forefront of Botox techniques and have all injected a great many patients. Sometimes, a magazine article uses me or one of these other doctors as the quoted expert. However, more often than not the "expert" is someone who does not do a lot of Botox, doesn't even really understand Botox, but has paid a PR person rather large sums of money to be the person who gets quoted in the press. The final goal of this person is obviously to draw in more patients since he's not getting enough referrals otherwise.

I would tell you also to beware of the doctor whose own hype is over the top. Avoid physicians with outrageous Web site claims or whose staff makes outrageous claims like "He has never given a patient a droopy eyelid." If that is true, he probably has not done much Botox either. Another trend that is neither good nor bad but mostly comical is the over-the-top name of the office. The office is often called the Anytown Institute of Plastic Surgery or the Academy of Advanced Dermatologic Sciences. Please. These places are only doctors' offices. I call my office "my office." Web site names are a different story. Their goal is to attempt to draw traffic. Most of the good names were taken in the mid-'90s when the domain names were registered. A lot of the names are way over the top. About a year ago, while working on this book, I went through the process of registering the domain name www.thebotoxbook.com. While doing so, I plugged in all sorts of other names that had already been taken. Guess what was not taken—"natural plastic surgery." I thought that would have been registered a long time ago. It has always been my overriding practice philosophy to have my patients look as natural as possible. But in this day of wild hype and overdone wind-tunnel facelifts, I guess no one wanted the word *natural*.

If you don't have any friends who have had Botox yet, I would recommend contacting either the the American Academy of Dermatology (888-462-DERM), the American Society of Plastic Surgeons (888-4 PLASTIC), or the American Society for Aesthetic Plastic Surgery (888-ASAPS 11) (plastic surgeons who specialize in cosmetic plastic surgery). These societies can refer you to physicians in your area who have been certified by either the American Board of Dermatology (313-874-1088) or the American Board of Plastic Surgery (215-587-9322). You can also check out a short list of doctors that I refer patients to. The list can be found on the Web site www.thebotoxbook.com or www.findabotox expert.com. As a disclaimer, I cannot guarantee that you'll be happy with your results by these injectors. What I can tell you is that these physicians are thought to be at the forefront of their field or at the very least are board-certified or have attended one of my lectures or live demonstrations.

6

THE PROCEDURE

Narrowing the Margin for Error

So now you've decided to go through with it and have selected a physician. Next comes the consultation. Usually, since a Botox injection is a fairly quick procedure, the consultation and injection are scheduled together. However, if your physician appears rushed, does not answer your questions to your satisfaction, or you just have a bad feeling about that person, do not go ahead with the injection. High-pressure sales belong in the used-car lot and *not* in the office of a reputable physician. Don't be coerced by the doctor or his office staff who tells you that he is so busy that you won't be able to get another appointment until the next millennium. You wouldn't want that appointment anyway. If your doctor says that you need Botox, I would think twice about that person. Nobody *needs* Botox. At least not cosmetically. Your doctor should take the time to examine your face, both in repose and in animation. He or she should be able to tell you about the risks particular to your face and the specific areas that you are having injected. If you do not feel comfortable, go no further. This is America. You're certainly allowed to leave the office, think it over, and if at a later date change your mind, schedule an injection. Over the years, I've had many people who come in for an initial consultation but then lose their nerve. So it throws a little speed bump in the middle of my office hours that day. So what. It's no big deal. The great majority of these people have come back at a later time and had me inject them. I've even had a few patients that come in for their consultation but chicken out at the last second. They then recommended me to their friends. Then they see their friends' result, and reschedule their procedure! I wonder if their friends were informed that they were being used as guinea pigs.

The one complication that no one wants is ptosis, or drooping, of the eyelid after an injection. This happens for one of two reasons. In the first, somehow the physician injects Botox into the wrong muscle—the wrong muscle being the thin wispy muscle in your eyelid that raises it. Over ten years, I can tell you that I've never seen that happen to one of my several thousand patients. Knowing anatomy, being careful, and taking a few certain basic steps to prevent seeping of the Botox should make this occurrence extraordinarily rare. The second reason—and I think the more common one—that this happens has to do with the variability in muscular anatomy and muscular strength between patients. In some patients the little eyelid muscle is a little too weak to do the job on its own. Usually this weakness is very minor, just a question of degree. Most patients with this problem don't realize that they have this weakness. That is because other muscles around the eyelid can compensate for this weakness and help the eyelid muscle to raise the eyelid. The muscle that helps it is the forehead muscle. The problem is, these are muscles that are weakened by well-placed Botox injections. There is no surefire way to 100 percent identify those patients that are high risk for developing a drooping eye after Botox injections, but there are clues to this weakness. Your injector should search for these clues prior to treatment. If you are at high risk, he should certainly inform you of this fact. There are also different techniques to inject the high-risk patient to decrease the risk of eyelid ptosis.

Some of these patients have been included in the photos. The patient in Figs. 9 through 14 has a slightly weak muscle in her left eyelid. This was recognized before injection. The injection pattern in her forehead was altered. If she had had a "routine" forehead injection the odds are overwhelming that she would have had a very droopy left eyelid afterward. Instead, not only did her lid not droop, I was actually able to make it better by lifting her left brow and pulling up on that left eyelid.

The woman in Figs. 43 through 46 also was a setup for disaster. Her left lid was already very low. By giving her a one-sided Botox browlift, a complication was avoided and her appearance improved.

The biggest risk factor is if you've had a droopy eyelid on a previous injection that was given by a pretty good injector. I used to say that any previous droopy lid experience was a strong risk factor. Not anymore. With the tremendous increase in Botox injections across the country, there has also been a tremendous increase in injectors who lack either the training, patience, or ability to become proficient injectors. Because of this, it seems to me that the incidence of a droopy eyelid due to getting Botox into the wrong muscle is inching up, not down.

If you do find a good injector, stick with that person. I know that the more I inject my patients, the better my results are. Not huge differences, but subtle little nuances that my patients appreciate. Do not jump around from physician to physician based on price or advertising. You get what you pay for.

Now you have decided to see what Botox can do for you and you have chosen a physician. You are excited and maybe a little bit nervous about what will happen next. Excited because maybe Botox can eliminate some of the fine lines and pesky problems around your face that have started to bother you lately. Nervous because you've already heard about its creating a droopy eyelid, which can sometimes follow an injection. To help avoid this and other problems, there are some things that your doctor will need to know. You might as well think these through beforehand so that you're ready to answer some questions in the office.

- Have you ever been diagnosed with a neuromuscular disorder such as myasthenia gravis or Lambert-Eaton syndrome? If you have, Botox injections are not for you.
- Do you currently have an infection being treated with antibiotics? Certain antibiotics preclude the use of Botox.
- Is there a possibility that you may be pregnant?
- Are you trying to become pregnant? I do not inject patients who are nursing, pregnant, or trying to become pregnant.
- Have you ever had any plastic surgery operations?
- Have you had any surgery at all to your face?
- Have you had Botox injections before?
- If you have had Botox infections, to what areas?
- When was the last time you had a Botox injection?
- Have you ever had a droopy eyelid after Botox injection?
- Did the droopy eyelid happen every time you had an injection or was it just one time?
- How long did the droopy eyelid take to get better?
- Are you happy with all the areas that you've had injected previously?
- Did your eyebrows appear droopy after your injections?

These are all important questions for trying to fine-tune your initial results with a new injector. If your physician doesn't want to know the answers to these questions maybe you need to find another injector.

Other questions aren't so obvious.

- Have you ever had what people sometimes called a sleepy eye at any time in your life?
- If you had a sleepy eye, did it go away on its own?
- Did you ever see a doctor for this sleepy eye condition?
- Are you the kind of person who shows a lot of upper eyelid while your eyes are open?
- Did anyone ever tell you have "bedroom eyes"?

- If you haven't gotten enough sleep or had a long, brutal day, do your eyelids ever feel extra heavy?
- Does one of your eyelids ever actually droop under these conditions?

If so, you may be predisposed to developing a droopy eyelid. Developing a droopy eyelid doesn't mean that Botox injections won't work really well for you. But it's important to give your doctor all this information.

This is critical information to help your doctor avoid giving you a droopy eyelid. As I said before, sometimes a droopy lid happens when Botox is injected carelessly or into the wrong muscle. Unfortunately, I think this is happening more and more as Botox becomes ever more popular. With the new stampede of patients following the FDA approval, more and more physicians are just starting out using Botox. This includes physicians of many specialties who may or may not have been trained in the anatomy of the different muscles and their different functions throughout the face. I think for most experienced injectors, injecting the wrong muscle is a rare occurence. I think the key is that some people have a weakness in their eyelid-raising muscle of which they are not aware. People are often unaware of the small asymmetries in their face. That's because they've been there all their lives or have slowly increased over many years. Eyelid asymmetry and eyelid level is one of the biggest tipoffs toward a predisposition to developing an eyelid droop. You cannot really help your injector with his examination of your face, but you can certainly alert him to this possibility by giving a thorough and accurate medical history.

Another problem that can follow Botox injections is bruising. Certainly, bruising is not nearly so bad as a droopy lid, but it is all a question of degree. Any time any one of us has a needle pierce our skin, a bruise is a possibility. A bruise is simply blood that has escaped from its blood vessel and is trapped within the tissues of the body. Sometimes that blood vessel has been crushed, as when a blunt object squeezes your soft tissues and skin against the bone underneath. This is similar to a boxer getting hit in the skin around his eye and turning black-and-blue.

This mechanical trauma crushes the small blood vessels, allowing the blood within them to escape and drift out into the skin, fat, and muscle of the face. We see this as a bruise. Sometimes, the blood vessels are cut, as when someone cuts himself on a piece of glass or tin can and a bruise develops. Fortunately, the needle is a relatively small sharp object. Occasionally, even a small needle will hit a blood vessel. Hopefully, it won't be a large blood vessel. Any area of the face can bruise after injection but some areas are more prone to bruising than others. In my practice, the area most susceptible to bruising is the crow's feet/lower eyelid area. Despite the fact that the skin in these areas is very thin and delicate, it often contains many fairly large blood vessels and veins. Sometimes the skin is so thin that these blood vessels can be seen through it. I always use a very bright light when injecting these areas so I can avoid touching the visible vessels with the tip of the needle. Some patients are so veiny in this area that I have to give them many mini injections with the needle despite the fact that I'm only putting a small dose of Botox into the area. Why? So I can dance around between the spiderweb of small veins that I'm looking at below the surface of the skin, avoiding touching them and avoiding giving my patient a big black eye. If the patient has been adequately prepared and is not taking any medications that thin the blood and the visible blood vessels are avoided, any resulting bruise is usually the size of a pencil eraser and is easily concealed with makeup.

Besides looking carefully for blood vessels, another trick that works very well is icing my patients. Most patients think the ice is for their comfort. That's only part of it. The ice also does two other things for me. One, it helps to keep the Botox where I put it. And two, it helps to decrease the chance of a bruise. Even if a bruise occurs, it helps to minimize its size. Patients who are concerned about their appearance do not want a black eye no matter how temporary it is. Icing the skin constricts these blood vessels before I put the needle into the skin. This makes it much less likely that one of these blood vessels will be touched by the sharp needle. Why I first began doing Botox injections, I did not routinely ice my patients and my bruising rate was approximately 10 percent. With careful icing before injection, I was able to cut my bruising to 4 percent. But the key is to apply the ice beforehand. If you just use ice after the injection, the horse is already out of the barn. After the injection, a blood vessel has either already been hit or not been hit. Icing after the injection will not help to prevent a bruise. Granted, if you are developing a bruise, icing afterward can help to limit the size and extent of the bruise. But you've already got the bruise. Bruising can happen anywhere that you receive an injection. But it is more prevalent around the eyes even if all the visible blood vessels beneath the skin are avoided. The reason is that muscles have a tremendous blood supply relative to the skin and fat around them. For Botox to work at its best, it should be injected into the muscle. Even the small muscles have pretty large, deep blood vessels that you cannot see. And so if you're a good injector and nearly always have the tip of your needle in the muscle when injecting, you're going to hit a blood vessel once in a while. At least hopefully it's a shriveled blood vessel due to the ice. The muscle around the eyes is very superficial. There is not a lot of fat covering it, and the skin is almost tissue-paper thin. Contrast that to the muscle between the eyes. This muscle is very deep, sitting on top of the bone. There's a fair amount of fat and very thick skin on top of it. If you hit a tiny blood vessel here and a small amount of blood escapes, you probably won't even be able to see a bruise. It will still be there and maybe this area will be a little bit sore to the touch for a week or so, but it won't be visible. Around the eyes, almost every drop of blood outside a blood vessel is visible as a bruise.

What can you do to prevent bruising? Actually, more than your doctor can. And that starts with your preparation for your injection two weeks before it actually happens. Many common medications thin the blood. What that means is they actually decrease the ability of your blood to form a clot. Besides the cells in the blood that transport oxygen to the different organs and the cells in the blood that fight infection, the blood also contains platelets. Platelets have many functions, but perhaps their most important is to begin the formation of a clot once a blood vessel has been damaged. This clot helps to seal the blood vessel and minimize leakage of blood. Many over-the-counter medications interfere with the platelets' work. They prevent or greatly reduce a platelet's ability to seal a leak. The medication that does this most powerfully is perhaps the most widely used medication in the world, aspirin. This permanently prevents your platelets from being able to start a blood clot. Other medications that interfere with your platelets include the nonsteroidal anti-inflammatory drugs such as Motrin, Aleeve, Nuprin, Naprosyn, ibuprofen, Advil, and so forth. How strict am I about not letting my patients have any of these medications before injection? Not at all. That is up to the patient. Your body re-forms and replenishes its supply of platelets about every two weeks. Therefore, to be sure that there are no effects left over from these medications, they should not be taken for two weeks before injection. But lots of patients use these medications very frequently. So would I refuse to inject the patient who has taken a couple of tablets of ibuprofen ten days ago? No. The small increase in the chance of bleeding will not adversely affect the Botox injection. In other words, the injection will work just as well with some of these medications on board as without. I am very strict about these medications before surgery. It would be foolhardy to do a facelift, rhinoplasty, or eyelid surgery without the patient's being 100 percent able to form clots. It would make the surgery not only messy but actually dangerous for the patient. An injection is not surgery. These drugs won't interfere with the final result. They will, however, increase your risk of bruising. The only patients that I'm very strict with regarding their medications are on-camera performers. These people cannot afford to have a bruise on their face while shooting. If they're shooting a scene over two days and one day they have a bruise and the other day they don't, there will be a continuity error in the film. I don't want to be blamed for this. So does this means that if you have had a few Advil ten days ago that you might as well keep taking some right up until the morning of your injection? No. Everything is relative, a question of degree here. Not having any of these medications for two days is better than taking them right up until the time of injection. But anyone who takes some within two weeks of their injection should realize that they are at a slightly higher risk for bruising than if they hadn't done so. This is why Tylenol (acetaminophen) is such a popular medication. It does not affect your platelets and so does not affect your clotting ability. For any aches or pains prior to surgery or injections, Tylenol is the medication of choice. If you look closely you can see a faint bruise across the bridge of the nose of the patient in Figs. 2 and 4. She had taken ibuprofen a few days before her injection.

But these are all relative risks. Some patients take a baby aspirin every day. Sometimes, this is something that they just heard was good for them, so based on friends' advice or a magazine article, they do it. Some patients have been put on an aspirin a day on the advice of their cardiologist. I take the second patient a bit more seriously. Everything has to do with relative risk. If people are taking an aspirin a day to help keep their heart healthy, I think that is more important than an increased risk of bruising after Botox injections. I do not tell these people to stop taking their aspirin. It's just common sense. By the way, the whole reason that some heart patients are told to take aspirin is because it thins the blood and makes it less likely to clot. That is because people with coronary artery disease are predisposed to having a clot form in the blood vessels that bring oxygen to their heart. So it is the same anticlotting effect of aspirin that they're looking for in the first place. That's why it works. If you're taking aspirin every day on the advice of your cardiologist because you're at an increased risk of heart attack that takes priority.

Initial and Ongoing Costs

Now you have decided on your injector and have prepared yourself mentally and physically for your injections. How much is this going to cost? Your initial fee will be for your consultation and perhaps your first set of Botox injections. Usually, the initial consultation and injections are done at the same appointment. Typically, when this is done, there is no separate charge for the consultation and the fee is solely for the Botox injections. But if you are nervous, or just want to think it over and you do not go through with your injections on the first appointment, you should expect to pay the consultation fee. This is not to punish you. This fee covers your doctor's time and evaluation of your face and neck concerning potential Botox injections whether or not you actually ever go through with them. Your fee will depend on how many areas you have injected. Depending on where you live, and whom you go to see, an average range for injections is from $500 to $1,500. When I first began doing Botox injections, I charged my patients a flat rate no matter how many areas I injected or how much Botox I used. I did this because I thought many patients would benefit from use of Botox in areas other than the standard areas of the frowning muscles, worry lines, and crow's feet. Many patients were initially surprised when I told them I thought it would work well in their neck, smile lines, or chin. I did not charge any additional fees for these areas because I didn't want it to seem as though I were selling them or trying to drive up their bill. A few years ago I changed that policy, not because I gave in to the dark side and turned to high-pressure sales, but because of the realities of my practice. Due to my unusual flat rate policy, my practice became top-heavy with patients having five or six areas injected. Only rarely did I have patients who had only one or two areas to inject. So I changed my fees accordingly.

The other question is how much this will cost over many years. The initial effects of Botox usually last from between three to six months. Usually, excellent results are seen for the first three months while the weakening of the muscles is in full effect. For the next three months the patient experiences diminishing returns as more and more muscular function returns to the face. Some patients schedule their appointments two and a half to three months apart, or call requesting to be seen on the first day that their motion returns. Some patients squeeze everything they can out of their injections and return every six or seven months. But on the average, most patients return about every four months. If you are having a few areas done and doing them every four months, you can probably expect to pay about $3,000 a year for your Botox injections. Some patients feel that they can put off a facelift or browlift or eyelid surgery with Botox, and since initially it is cheaper, they feel that economically this is a sound judgment. But they are mistaken on two counts. Firstly, Botox is usually not a replacement for surgery. These surgical operations mostly deal with loose hanging skin and fat and occasionally muscle. Botox will not do anything for hanging skin and fat. Although Botox can elevate the brows, it does not do it in the same way as a browlift. These two are not exactly equivalent. Also, just because someone has a browlift, that doesn't mean that the person would never benefit from future Botox injections. They do different things. So, if someone tries to put off a browlift for economic reasons for five years, using Botox, that person may spend $15,000 to avoid a $5,000 operation.

Prep Talk

Before you meet with your physician during the consultation, you should think about what you are going to say and ask. You should be prepared to discuss with your physician the areas of your face that most bother you. Be prepared to not only discuss *what* bothers you but *how* it bothers you. For instance, some people are bothered by lines on their face when they are at rest and some patients are more bothered by the lines that come out when their face is fully animated. Some patients actually like the crow's feet around their eyes. Everyone is different. You've already prepared your medical history with regard to your face and Botox injections in particular. You should also be prepared to ask some questions. Sometimes making a short list so that you don't forget anything is a good idea. That's just being prudent. No doctor should mind a short list of questions that pertain to a procedure they may be doing on a patient. However, it is best to avoid bringing a legal pad filled with two hundred questions that you would like to ask your doctor. That is probably not such a great idea. Some pertinent sample questions:

- How long have you been injecting Botox?
- How many Botox injections do you perform in a day, a week, a month?
- Do you feel comfortable injecting the nontraditional areas of the face and neck?
- How often do your patients get a droopy eyelid or bruise?

Also be prepared to discuss how weakened you want your muscles to be in a particular area. For instance:

- Would you mind not being able to frown at all?
- Would you mind not being able to wiggle your eyebrows?
- How important is lifting the eyebrows a bit to you?
- If you had to choose between having a smoother forehead or higher eyebrows, which would you pick?

One other thing. If you want your physician to really get a good sense of your wrinkles, skin, and motion do not walk into his examination room with all your makeup on. Makeup is great because it conceals these things that we want hidden. Since this is what you are being treated for you should not want to conceal these things from your doctor.

From my own perspective, I like it when patients have thought about their consultation in advance and done a little homework. While patients are discussing their problem areas and their concerns with me, I'm listening but also studying their face. While the patients are telling me what areas they would like to improve, I'm thinking which areas I would like to improve on their face and neck. As long as there is a fair amount of overlap between the two, I'm certain that patient satisfaction will be high. I do not inject every patient that I see for a Botox consultation. Sometimes the patient's wishes are so far apart from what I think would be a good aesthetic improvement that I decline. I feel other patients are looking for an unachievable result. This is an extremely subjective thing. Several years ago, I had a patient who asked for her money back. She said that she did not notice any change after her Botox injections. I told

her that I disagreed and thought that she had a very nice change and I
took a few pictures of her on that second visit. She called and left an
angry message with my receptionist the next week but never returned to
the office. When I saw her before- and after-photos, I was stunned. Not
only did she have a good result, she had one of the best results that I've
ever achieved. Despite the fact that her lines were fairly deep when I
saw her beforehand, her frown lines, crow's feet, and smile lines were
nearly totally eliminated in her after-photos despite a normal appearance. Yet in her mind, she saw no improvement. Patients often carry a
mental image of themselves that was imprinted in their mind ten or
twenty years previously. It's important to try to figure out who these
patients are before injection. After all, the whole point of these injections
is not just an objective improvement in appearance or wrinkle reduction.
The entire point is helping patients to feel better about themselves. And
if that's not going to happen, it's not worth doing the injection.

This brings me to a question that I'm often asked by other injectors.
In fact, at the Botox launch party to celebrate their FDA approval in
New York, I was asked this question by some well-known injectors who
do a lot of Botox. They wanted to know that since I had a reputation as
someone who prefers a normally moving face to the mask face without
any lines, how I handled patients who wanted more weakening with
fewer lines than I wanted to give them. This is a rather simple yet common problem that I handle differently depending on the patient. But it
also depends on the degree of disagreement. If I really feel a new patient
wants to have almost no expression and wants to eliminate every wrinkle
on her face, I decline to inject that person. Period. Usually, patients will
accept this. Sometimes they become a little bit upset, at which time I
look them straight in the eye and tell them that I don't feel that what I
could do for them would make them happy. They generally accept that
and leave without a fuss. Why would patients insist on a procedure that
would leave them disappointed with the results? The next question is,
how I deal with an established patient with the same problem. If I've
seen the patient for a few visits, and she wants a little more weakening,
I think that's okay. Again, this is not permanent procedure. Slight over-

weakening for someone who is fully aware of what that means, and who I think is a reasonable person with their head on straight, is okay by me. If that same patient keeps coming back to me for touch-ups after every injection with the goal of not moving at all, that's another story. Typically, I will give the patient the additional Botox injection at no charge. I do not want the patient to be angry. However, I will also tell her that this degree of weakening, or outright paralysis, is not part of my practice philosophy. I then tell her that for her next injection, she would be better off going to a different physician. From the looks of some faces I see in restaurants and walking down the street, there is no shortage of physicians in New York who like to wipe every last bit of expression from their patients' faces. That usually handles that problem. Then again, there is the A-list patient. Maybe doctors aren't supposed to have favorite patients, but we all do. They are people who besides being your patients have also become your friends, and many have been with your practice since the beginning. First maybe I did their eyelids, then a few years later a little liposuction, then I have operated on their spouse or siblings. These are people that I like and I look forward to seeing their names on my daily schedule. Despite how well you get along, there's always room for a difference of opinion. And sometimes even these patients want to be a little more paralyzed than I want to make them. For these patients, I have a different solution. I agree to inject them a bit more strongly, more along the lines of what they desire after a little discussion. I tell them that they may not look so natural with a little more Botox on board, but if they still want it, I give it to them. But as they are leaving I tell them that the only reason I did it was because they are such good patients and that I would like to continue to take care of them so I have one favor to ask of them. Although I will continue to inject them in this fashion if they desire, I respectfully ask that they never tell anyone that I'm their injector. Usually, they look a little taken aback. I politely explain to them that I think they'd look a lot better with a little less weakening in their face. I also explain that my reputation is very important to me and I do not want to be known as the doctor that wipes all the expression from his patients' faces. I have worked very hard to build my practice over the last decade. And it is successful. And while I have a nice office and caring staff, I realize at the end of the day that all I really have is my name and reputation. Not always with the next injection but usually sometime down the road, this patient will tell me to maybe try a little bit less Botox and that maybe a little extra expression accompanied by a few extra lines aren't so bad after all.

Injection Time

The patient has been examined, her history taken, risks have been explained, and she's given her informed consent. Now it is time to actually do the injection. The patient has probably already removed her makeup if she is wearing any. If not, I remove it at this time. Sometimes my staff will stop a patient and ask her to remove her makeup and wash her face before entering the exam room. A frequent response is "I'm not wearing any" or "I just washed my face." Then I spend a minute or two removing her makeup prior to injection. I'm not sure why this is. I think that for some women, it takes so long to properly apply it that they don't want to remove it in case they do not go through with the injection. Some do not want to be without makeup for the ten-foot walk from the powder room to the exam room. But if you insist on your doctor examining you with makeup on, you should realize that it is a less than ideal examination. After removing the makeup, I recline the patient back to an almost recumbent position. I think one of the fallacies about Botox injections that is often spouted over and over again by injectors is that the patient must be in an upright position so it won't "seep down" into other muscles. I don't see any reason for that. I've always placed my patients almost flat on the examining chair.

After disinfecting the skin with alcohol, I begin to ice them. For a while, I had patients cooling their own faces with ice packs. Unfortunately, I don't think many of them did a good job. While waiting, instead of applying the ice packs, they would be reading a magazine. I didn't blame them. But you cannot read a magazine with an ice pack over your eyes. And while my office runs close to schedule (we do not double-book patients) I certainly have waited for long periods in another doctor's exam room with the door closed. You have no idea when that door will open. I would be bored too. When I ice my patients down, it is almost painful for them. I apply the ice directly and with some gentle pressure to the skin. One question I'm asked frequently is "What is that you're putting on me?" When I tell them that it is a regular ice cube, some patients don't believe it. They say that it feels too cold. The reason it feels so cold is that it's being applied with some pressure, since I'm trying to get the cold to penetrate through the skin down into the muscle and constrict those pesky blood vessels.

After icing, I begin with the injections. Once the patients are lying on the table, I ask them to close their eyes. I also talk very softly for several minutes to the patients in an attempt to relieve their anxieties. I explain to them step-by-step what's going on, through their makeup removal, skin cleansing, and icing. I assure them that I am not going to sneak up on them and inject them unexpectedly with the needle. They are also asked to concentrate on their breathing. I ask them to open their mouths and take slow, deep, regular breaths through the mouth. I try to get them to focus on their breathing and tell them not to lose that focus, even when I'm doing the injections. This helps lead to relaxed patients who will not strain or hold their breath when I begin to inject. It also helps to reduce the risk of headache and bleeding and bruising. By not having the patient's heart hammering during the injections, it also helps to keep the Botox where I precisely place it with my needle. I nearly always start with the frowning muscles, since most patients feel that is the most painful area. The patients are asked to keep their eyes closed, and I actually lift up on the eyebrow that I am starting with and squeeze the skin fairly firmly against the bone that forms the top of the eye socket. This helps to form a physical barrier against the Botox possibly seeping around this bone toward the area of the muscle that raises the eyelid. The patient is then asked to make several expressions so that I can visualize the muscles beneath the skin and start my injections. I always give my patients a short break between areas just to catch their breath. They are asked to refocus their energies on their slow, easy breathing during the quiet resting times between areas. I will usually move to the forehead next, followed by the crow's feet, and then down through the areas of the face from top to bottom. Patients sometimes get a bit nervous between areas, so it is always reassuring to tell them that the worst, most painful area has already been done. With most injections, there's very little bleeding. But sometimes a bit of blood will come out when I remove the needle. That is a sign to me that a small blood vessel has probably been poked by the needle. I quickly apply pressure and ice to this area and hold it steady for several minutes. I do this even though I have already broken the blood vessel. With firm pressure and ice usually I can limit the extent of the bruise and in thicker skin areas actually prevent a visible bruise from forming. Although it takes an extra five minutes or so, I certainly think it is worth it to the patient.

Sometimes patients tell me they can hear a light crackling noise during their injections. This is normal. Each of the tiny muscles injected is covered by a thin membrane resembling a sausage casing. This is what can crackle when it gets swollen with the Botox.

A question that nervous patients often ask is how many injections are they actually going to have. That is a question I cannot answer beforehand. When I examine the different areas of a patient's face, I'm making an educated judgment as to the total Botox dose for that area. I then load my syringe with that amount of Botox and try to visualize the muscles beneath the skin as the patient makes several expressions. I put the Botox where I think it is most needed to control wrinkling, motion, and eyebrow shape. Sometimes there will be two pinpricks in the forehead and sometimes fifteen. The strange thing is, due to the effect of the ice and quickness of each injection, patients are often unsure of how many injections they have actually gotten. Very often I will do five small quick injections along one eyebrow and the patient will ask me if that was one. The needle is very small, and the properly prepared skin feels only a slight pinch. Most of the pain comes from the medication being injected into the small muscle, which feels more like a dull ache than sharp pain.

So several quick injections very often feel like a single four- or five-second injection to the patient.

Another question patients often have at this time concerns numbing creams. These became popular in the early to mid-'90s. There are several excellent preparations on the market, such as EMLA, Elamax, Topicaine, and Betacaine. All of these medications penetrate into the skin. They contain local anesthetics that help to numb the skin. The problem is, they don't penetrate very deeply, certainly not all the way through thick skin, through the fat, and into a deep muscle. If patients request them or have them I don't mind if they put them on an hour before their appointment. That's how long they take to work. When properly applied, they are not deleterious. In general, I think they do not really do much good except for the crow's feet area with its very thin skin and superficial muscle.

Immediate Aftercare

My post-injection instructions are very simple. They are also based on years of experience and some science. The instructions that I read in magazines from other "experts" are very often a source of amusement in my office. Just as good are some instructions patients have told me that other doctors have given them previously. I have heard instructions such as: you can't tie your shoes for six hours (what happens if your shoes are untied and you don't have a personal valet to tie them for you? Are you supposed to trip and cut your head open?); you cannot lie down for six hours (if you can lie down during your injection, why can't you lie down after it?); you can't read a book for six hours (as if using and moving your eyes was somehow going to magnetically suck the Botox out of your head and make it run down into your eye muscles); you need to wear a foam rubber collar or scarf around your neck for four hours to make sure your head doesn't tip down (just picture that); no exercising for twenty-four hours (why?). My instructions are fairly simple. No heavy lifting, straining, or raising your heart rate for two hours. You can bend down if you need to but I prefer it if you bend more with your knees and less with your waist. That's it. No other instructions. When you go to your physician, whom you have selected and hopefully trust, you should follow his or her instructions.

When Botox is injected into the muscle, it needs to bind itself to the outside of the nerve to start to work. Studies show that this takes about one and a half hours. So for that one and a half hours, I don't want to increase the circulation to that area to "wash away" the Botox from where it was injected. Since it has stuck to the nerve after about an hour and a half, that's when I lift my restrictions. I round this up to two hours just to be safe. Straining, heavy lifting, and bending your head forward at the waist can increase the circulation to these areas. But after two hours I see no reason not to resume normal activity. When I first started using Botox, we didn't know that it bound to the nerve after one and a half hours and so my initial instructions were the same except that I used to tell people to follow them for six hours. About eight years ago, when several patients had told me that they had forgotten, gone to the gym, jogged, and so forth without any ill effects, I dropped my time restriction to four hours. But for the last two years I have had a two-hour limitation.

For the patient with a little bleeding or bruising, holding ice to that spot afterward can help to minimize the appearance of the bruise. When I do get a bruise, the overwhelming majority are the size of a pencil eraser or less. I think this is mostly due to icing and pressure as soon as bleeding is noted. But bruising is unusual. The vast majority of my patients will have only a few small red dots on their face when the injection is completed. These red dots usually take only about fifteen minutes to go away. Patients can reapply their makeup before leaving the office.

Patients often ask me how they should adjust their skin care routine when getting Botox injections. Basically, I tell them they don't need to. Patients who are using Retin-A, glycolic acid, vitamin C, Kinerase, or other skin care products can continue their routines around the Botox injection. I would not recommend that a patient have a facial or micro-dermabrasion immediately after injection. These two therapies increase the local circulation to the area; therefore there is a slight chance of changing the results of the injection by disturbing the precise placement of Botox. For the past two years, however, I have allowed patients to have a light "lunchtime" peel, facial, or microdermabrasion at the same appointment and as long as the skin care comes first. I have seen no adverse effects from these therapies when done before, not after, the Botox injection. In fact, I encourage my patients to have this done. Proper skin care, including avoidance of the sun, no smoking, moderate alcohol intake, medications shown to reduce the signs of aging of the skin, as well as microdermabrasion, all complement and improve the results that you see after Botox injection. That's because these therapies are aimed at rejuvenating the skin. Botox is aimed at relaxing the muscle, which then stops beating up the skin. But anything that helps the skin to actually recover from its past abuses is very synergistic and adds greatly to the result that you can get with Botox. Many patients have been told that after Botox injections it is imperative that they stay out of the sun. While I certainly don't recommend sun exposure for anyone, I have not noticed any particular ill effects of sun exposure on Botox injections per se. But you are damaging your skin.

A PATIENT'S VIEWPOINT
Our History: His, Mine, and Botox's

It was during the mid-1990s that I heard the word Botox used for the very first time. While that doesn't seem so long ago, added perspective comes from remembering that the hot topic in plastic surgery at that time was the breast implant scare, not the newest treatment for eliminating wrinkles. Back then, Kane was a junior attending surgeon at the prestigious Manhattan Eye, Ear and Throat Hospital and I clearly remember him going on and on about a new cosmetic application for what I understood to be a diluted form of botulism. I remember this, specifically, not because I had any great interest in

Botox, but because of Kane's excitement and because I both liked and related to the pioneering aspect of the story.

Kane, truly one of the most intellectually curious people I've ever known, had for years been obsessed, specifically, with the effect Bell's palsy had on its victims. As he explained to me then, the disease caused paralysis on one side of the face. As a result, the side of the face that was affected was left looking smooth and uncreased.

This obsession came into play when Kane and his Program Director at Manhattan Eye, Ear and Throat, Bill Nolan, were shooting the breeze—professionally speaking, of course—with Dr. Richard Lisman, "an eye guy" at the hospital. The "eye guys" had for years been using Botox to relax (read: paralyze) muscles that caused crossed eyes. What if, Kane wondered, as with crossed eyes, you could temporarily paralyze facial muscles with Botox? Might this result in the same kind of smooth and unwrinkled skin found in patients who had Bell's palsy?

To say Kane was extremely excited about using Botox in this way would have been an understatement. To say that my enthusiasm matched his would have been an outright lie. First, there was the less than appetizing aspect of botulism (a connection that brought to mind bloated tin cans). Then, given all the talk of Bell's palsy and lazy eyes, well—I can't say I understood, or was drawn to, the innovation about which he was so obviously enthused.

Which is not to say that I wasn't profoundly intrigued by Kane's discoveries in his line of work. In fact, my interest was both personal and professional. On the personal front, Kane and I were, at that time, a couple. I took, and still do take, immense pride in his achievements. Though I teased him mercilessly about being the Doogie Houser of plastic surgery, it's no small feat that Kane finished his undergraduate and medical studies in an accelerated five years before going on to become the youngest plastic surgeon in the history of plastic surgery. This accomplishment is something that, to this day, Kane plays down. My feeling is that, in addition to its being impressive, this experience instilled in Kane the confidence to pioneer and tenaciously pursue ideas that others have at first found provocatively innovative. And Botox is just one case in point.

Professionally, my interests dovetailed with Kane's because of my job as a magazine editor. When we met, I was working on the newly launched In Style *magazine. Previously, I'd been the beauty editor at* Mirabella *and prior to that had, over the years, written and assigned stories covering new treatments and procedures in plastic surgery. And yet, I still didn't follow Kane when he described how Botox would evolve into a truly revolutionary weapon in the fight against aging.*

Leave it to Kane, though, who persisted. His personal goal at that time was amassing enough "before and after" photos so that he could deliver his paper on Botox and see it published in the Journal of Plastic and Reconstructive Surgery. *Where this task sounds easy and logical in theory, in practice it was daunting. First, most patients bolted at the initial description of Botox. Others took one look at the youngster proposing an unorthodox treatment and turned him down flat. Slowly, though, word spread about the results he'd had. As more patients came to the practice for Botox, more proof was committed to film.*

In terms of the history—his, mine, and Botox's—there were two seminal moments that I clearly remember. One was watching Kane deliver his first speech to a room filled with colleagues at the ASAPS conference at the Hilton Hotel in Manhattan. I've met enough plastic surgeons in my time to know that this group tends to be as skeptical as they are serious. As Kane delivered his speech, I couldn't help but realize that the crowd was rapt. Kane really did own the audience (remember Tom Cruise in Magnolia?*). The reason these doctors were entranced? They were empowered. They sat listening to information about just the thing that could change—that is, now, literally changing—the face of our culture.*

The other seminal moment came when a local station broadcast the first segment about the cosmetic use of Botox. The reporter definitely had her angle on the story—one that combined shock and disgust. I don't remember specifics from the script aside from her sign-off, which was: Let a plastic surgeon inject botulism into your face? Is this something you would do?

I don't know if the reporter has changed her view on Botox. I do know that since then I became one of the million or so people who has.

Me? A Candidate?

For all the talk about Botox, I'd never considered myself someone who needed it. First, given the personal nature of our relationship, I'd avoided becoming Kane's patient. As time went on, more and more friends told me how thrilled they were about what Kane had done for them. Still, I wasn't ready—physically or mentally—for anti-aging treatments more serious than good moisturizer and sunscreen.

Years later, when we were no longer a couple, I was sitting around with Kane when I jokingly said something about my being ready for Botox. Instead of joking with me, he said, "C'mere, stand by the window." Reverting to his serious, professional self, Kane looked at my forehead, asked me to make a smile, then a frown, and said, "Come see me in the office."

Sure, I'd known about Botox and spoken with Kane about it since its inception—but I was shocked. Shocked because this wasn't a clinical exchange, this was about me. You can spend your career writing and editing stories about antiaging treatments, but hitting the age when you become a candidate for those treatments, well, the polite distance of the purely theoretical is rudely replaced by the emotional wallop of ego.

Me a candidate? I just couldn't get over it. I was in my early thirties and it took me a little time to grasp the fact that yes, I was at "that age." Once I'd (sort of) come to terms with that part of the equation, I chose to focus my mind on what Kane had told me years before: Botox has preventative qualities. And so, I reasoned to myself, it was less that I really needed to have Botox immediately (though that would be a nice benefit). I was investing myself in keeping the inevitable creases and furrows at bay.

This is what I was still telling myself while sitting under the examining lamp in Kane's office on Manhattan's Upper East Side as he looked at my skin from behind a pair of magnifying glasses. In his calm, doctorly manner, Kane again asked me to smile, then relax, frown, then relax my face. He then ran his hand over my face, testing my skin's elasticity. After just a few minutes, he turned off the bright light and we began discussing his recommendations.

"I wouldn't do anything drastic," he said, "but there are areas where you'll see an immediate improvement." He then explained how he would

inject a very small amount of Botox to my forehead, which would lighten the crease that had begun to form there. He also suggested that he inject the space between my eyebrows where I was just starting to develop the fine lines that would develop into deeper creases with time.

Taking in this first dose of reality, I wanted first to know how it would affect the movement of muscles in my forehead.

Everyone, I assume, has unique and quirky physical traits that they become attached to over time. For some it's the ability to wiggle their ears, for others, it's curling their tongue. For me, it's all about the eyebrows. Because I can raise each brow individually, as well as the two together, I've been told my face is extremely expressive. I like that. (Not to mention, I'm a big hit entertaining the kids in my family under age ten). This wasn't something I was keen on giving up, vanity or not.

Kane assured me that I'd still be able to move my brows. He explained that while the crease in the center of my forehead would be smoother, the Botox wouldn't interfere or inhibit my range of expression. It would, though, prevent a furrow from forming between my eyebrows.

That was all I needed to hear. Growing older, the one thing I dreaded was the furrowed brow. Crow's feet, laugh lines, they didn't scare me. What I really wanted to avoid was aging into a look that made me appear angry or disapproving without ever being so.

Thus, my inhibition and (mild as it was) fear lost out to the big picture vision of what I wanted to look like. And that decision in itself was, on some level, incredibly empowering.

Is This Going to Hurt?

Honestly, the most painful part of the process was realizing that I'd reached an age where Botox had been recommended.

Making the decision to go forward, well, that was a leap of faith that, owing to the trust I had in my friend and doctor, didn't give me reason to hesitate.

The scariest moment? I can tell you this: the apprehension and anxiety that precede the injections are far, far worse than actually being injected.

In fact, signing the release allowing Kane to use Botox may have even been scarier. Until that moment, I had never imagined I'd willingly consent to having a known poison injected into my body.

That said, Kane allayed my fears by talking me through the entire procedure. Back in the chair, he told me that first he would lower the chair into a reclining—or what he joked was business class—position. For some reason, this had the effect of making me feel less anxious. Then, he cleaned my skin with alcohol.

Next, Kane said he would first numb the area with ice. But it felt uncomfortably cold, almost too cold to just be ice. This, he explained, was because he applied the ice with more force than I would have used on myself—the reason being that he wanted to have the freezing effect penetrate from the surface of the skin down into my muscles.

Kane then held my head in his hands and gently moved it from side to side until he found the angle that allowed him the best access and view of the portion of my face being injected. Once there, he studied my face closely, asking that I frown, then relax, smile, relax, raise my eyebrows and relax again. We repeated this cycle until Kane said I would soon feel a number of small pinpricks as he injected different areas. I did. It wasn't pleasant—but it wasn't what I'd call painful, either. A few of the pinpricks I barely felt at all. Other pinpricks were deeper, and I felt a low-level burning or stinging sensation.

Using a piece of gauze, Kane then applied gentle pressure across my eyebrows for what must have been a minute or two. He said this would allow me to catch my breath between areas, since he'd finished injecting between my brows and was about to wrap up with my forehead.

I don't know if it was the numbing effect the ice had had, or whether I'd steeled myself for pain that was out of proportion, but that it was over so quickly was news to me. Yes, I'd felt the pinpricks, but where, exactly, or how many there had been I couldn't tell you.

After the break, Kane again applied the ice and had me repeat the cycle of facial expressions I'd made earlier. This time, when I felt the pinpricks, it was, as Kane had said, less perceptible. This, he explained, was because the brow is more sensitive than the forehead area.

And that was my experience. For me it was less painful than a leg and bikini wax. And in the time it took for me to arrive at the analogy, the whole procedure was over.

Kane's next instructions were this: "Just for the next few hours, when you have to bend, bend at the knees, not the waist. And," he added, "skip the gym for today." Ah, what indulgence! Immediately, I promised to comply.

On my way out of the office, I couldn't resist a peek. I slipped into the washroom to check on the state of things. Just as Kane had said, no bruising, no bleeding, no signs at all save for a few minuscule red dots in the area he'd injected. All right, what's the deal, I couldn't help but wonder.

To recap: Big deal on the aging and ego front, less a big deal on the decision to do it front, no big deal on the actual injection front.

B Is for Benefit

That night, even though I could have, I didn't make plans to go out or have friends over. Instead, I watched and waited. Nothing. Nada. Nichts. It wasn't until two mornings later that I first saw results. And what I saw was amazing.

For all that Kane had pointed at the crease in my forehead, I really hadn't seen what he was talking about. Looking into the mirror forty-eight hours later, I finally realized what had been there—but only in contradiction to what was, or wasn't, there then. The skin on my forehead was smooth. Not completely, not to the point where it seemed taut or unnatural but, if it can be explained like this, where the skin looked less jagged.

The other thing that had changed were my eyebrows. Kane had explained that the Botox might cause them to seem raised. Try though I might to understand what he meant, I couldn't until I felt and saw it myself. My eyebrows sat ever so slightly higher than before. It wasn't something anyone would notice. In fact, I only began to notice when applying eyeshadow and seeing that the natural crease in my eyelids had lessened. Who knew? (Even though I had been told!) Fantastic.

Trying to raise each brow in my signature expression, nothing had changed. Each moved up and down; I could still move both in tandem. Then, as Kane had suggested, I attempted to frown. I still could, but the frown lines I made weren't nearly as severe.

It took a few hours to get used to the new sensations. Not that I would have known that if I hadn't been trying to move my face in some kind of test. By midday, I'd completely forgotten to make faces.

That, some four years ago, was my experience with Botox. Kane said that, on average, Botox lasts about six months. The results I saw were still in evidence some two years later. Two years later, had I not found myself waiting for Kane to finish with patients one night, I probably wouldn't have bothered having a touch-up for, well, who knows how long. As I was there, I thought, might as well—couldn't hurt. Now, that was two years ago. Would I consider another round of Botox? Only when necessary—and given the results I've seen, I can only say that when *remains a question still to be determined . . . sometime in the future.*

7

MAKING IT LAST

~~~~~~~~~~~~~~~~~~~
~~~~~~~~~~~~~~~~~~~

The Effect of Repeated Injections

There is sometimes a large misunderstanding on both the part of patients and physicians when it comes to the effect of repeated Botox injections. Back in 1997, I was on a panel presenting papers on Botox injections before a large group of plastic surgeons at the meeting of the American Society for Aesthetic Plastic Surgery. The expert moderator of the panel was asked a question about repeated injections. At that time, Botox was not a very common procedure for most plastic surgeons. The moderator stated that the effects of Botox over time typically diminish. For that reason, he was often forced to use more and more Botox to achieve the same effect. In my experience, that is exactly the opposite of what happens. I politely tapped on my microphone and completely disagreed with the speaker. It did not endear me to my senior plastic surgeons, but it was the right thing to do. Frankly, I'm not sure how rumors like this get started. I think sometimes that physicians think that one medication is analogous to another. They then derive incorrect conclusions based on a faulty analogy.

I've heard this same mistaken idea of building up a resistance to Botox being equated to developing a tolerance for narcotics. Because in either the hospitalized patient or the addict, repeated injections of narcotics will have less and less effect with time, requiring higher and higher doses for either pain relief or euphoria. But that is not how Botox works. The mechanism of action of the two drugs is different. Once a muscle is paralyzed, giving more and more Botox obviously doesn't make it more paralyzed. However, giving more and more narcotics provides the person more pain relief or euphoria.

But the biggest puzzle to me is how doctors who have been injecting Botox could say such a thing. Because even if they thought that things ought to work this way, clinically they don't. If they paid attention to their patients and how much motion they have, and how frequently they come in for a new set of injections, these doctors would realize that in the great majority of patients, the effect of Botox lasts longer and longer.

The reason for this can be seen in a different analogy, which is much closer to how Botox really works. Let's go back to the broken-arm analogy. Say you break your arm and it is put in a cast for three months. That is a long time for your muscles not to be able to move. During that time, your muscles get weaker and weaker due to strict inactivity. Well, the same thing happens with Botox. Although your facial muscles are not put in a cast, they are prohibited from moving. This makes them weaker. When your cast is off at the end of three months, you can move your arm again. But not the way you could before the cast was placed. Your muscles are now very weakened and it will probably take a few months of physical therapy and exercises to get your arm back in the shape it was before you broke it. The same holds true for the facial muscles. That's why even though the effect of Botox is gone after ten to twelve weeks, the effect it has on your muscles lasts for much longer.

Now, say, instead of going through rehabilitation and lifting weights, a cast is reapplied to the same arm. The muscles are going to get weaker again. But the starting point isn't the same. The starting point isn't with your muscles at full strength. The starting point is with your muscles already weakened. With that cast on for another three months your arm will be pathetically weakened. This is very similar to the effect of repeated Botox injections.

This effect is most commonly seen along the frown lines. That is because this is the one area that I feel comfortable—and most patients want this more than I do—paralyzing completely. When this is done over the course of several years, almost all patients in my practice see some long-term weakening of these muscles. This is not something to be feared. As was discussed in the section about frown lines, during most tried-and-true surgical procedures along the brow, these muscles are actually removed and thrown away. So a little permanent weakening here would not be such a bad thing after all. These frowning muscles have no purpose other than for facial expression. They are not necessary to open or close the eyes or perform any other function.

For some reason, not every patient realizes the benefits of long-term weakening of these muscles. I'm not completely sure why, but I have a hunch. Patients who tend to not see weakening over the long haul tend to be those with extremely expressive faces. Some of these patients are almost cartoonish when you compare them to most people as far as their facial animation goes. But they are in the minority. These people send lots of impulses down their nerves to their muscles. Even if Botox blocks 98 percent of those impulses so that the muscle has no visible motion, 2 percent of a lot of impulses is nothing to sneeze at.

The other thing that I have never seen is complete, total, irreversible atrophy of these muscles. In other words, I've never had a patient who has had so many Botox injections to the frown area that the person was never able to frown again. So this is a reversible atrophy. I think the reason can be found in the analogy to the facial paralysis patient. Muscles need to receive nerve impulses to command them to move. Without the impulse, there is no motion. Without any motion, the muscle will atrophy, wither, and die. So why don't patients who continually paralyze their frowning muscles induce these muscles to wither completely? I think the answer lies in the nerve-to-muscle connection. For the muscle to receive no impulses, there must be zero nerves telling it to move. That is a tall order. I think that even when a muscle appears to be completely paralyzed by Botox, it's probable that a few nerve fibers are still talking to it. The thing is, we don't see any motion because these few nerves talk to very few muscle fibers and so we cannot see any clinical motion. But on a microscopic scale, you probably do have a little motion. And these impulses and that motion is probably enough to keep the muscle alive. I'm sure this happens especially right before subsequent injections. Occasionally, but very rarely, do patients come back for reinjection before they have any motion in the frown area. They come back because their neck or chin or crow's feet wrinkles have returned and so the frown muscles get injected even though there is no apparent motion yet. I think that it is during the period immediately before injection that even though the muscle does not appear to be moving, some nerve fibers have reattached themselves to the muscle and give it just enough of a signal to keep it alive. These impulses are not enough to build the muscle up, so that is why it is weakened but never completely withered.

This makes sense when you compare Botox patients to facial paralysis patients. There are several reasons why patients can develop paralysis on one side of their face. Sometimes it can be due to a tumor pressing on a nerve and preventing it from telling the muscles to move. It can be from a car accident or other traumatic event or surgery that damages the nerves. Most frequently, however, it is due to Bell's palsy. This is a condition, sometimes preceded by a viral ailment, that suddenly results in full or partial paralysis of one side of the face. Usually, these patients gradually get better and quite often have full return of strength to that side of the face. Sometimes, for whatever reason, that doesn't happen and one side remains weakened compared to the other. The big question is when to surgically intervene in any of these patients. From looking at the scientific literature dealing with facial paralysis patients, it is apparent that time is of the essence. Basically, if a muscle on the paralyzed side of the face does not reestablish a connection to a nerve within one and a half to two years, that muscle will atrophy completely. In other words, reconnecting it to a nerve after this time will not do any good at all, as

Figures 69–74: This patient in her forties did not like the extra little creases she made below her mouth when smiling and saying certain sounds.

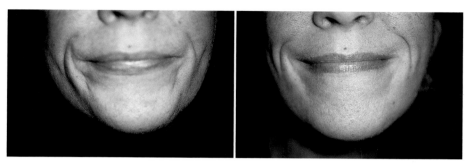

Figures 69 and 70: Smiling before and after. Note the disappearance of the extra little lines around and below the corners of the mouth despite a natural smile.

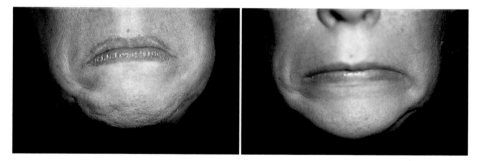

Figures 71 and 72: The patient used to ball up her chin (at left) when saying certain sounds, speaking forcefully, and chewing. She is unable to do so after injection.

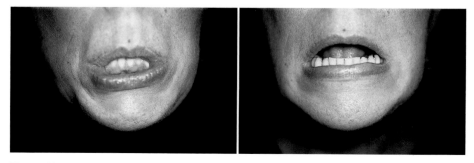

Figures 73 and 74: She was asked to show me her lower teeth in these photos. She can no longer make the sharp indentations below the corners of her mouth. This will prevent that area from prematurely aging.

Figures 75–78: The chin of the patient in these four photos had a classic cobblestone appearance.

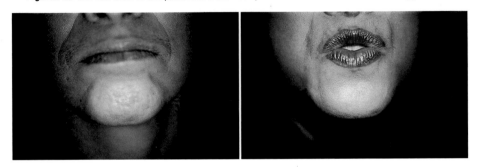

Figures 75 and 76: Closing her mouth tightly before and after injection.

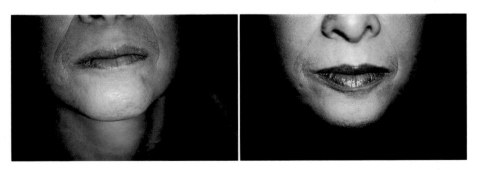

Figures 77 and 78: Even at rest this patient had dimpling of her chin, which is gone after her injection.

Figures 79–82: The neck before injection on left, after on right.

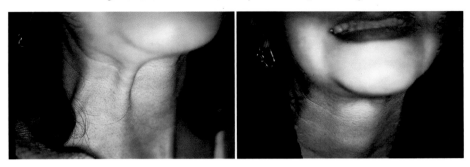

Figures 79 and 80: This woman in her late thirties was bothered by the cords beginning to run down her neck. They are markedly improved after injection. These cords are made of muscle and would have continued to pull down on her neck skin, prematurely aging it.

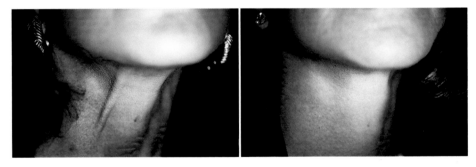

Figures 81 and 82: This woman in her late fifties has had a prior face and neck lift and has minimal excess skin of the neck. She has an excellent result.

Figures 83–88: This patient in her thirties had a history of prolonged sun exposure and smoking. After receiving regular injections for years, she did not have any for nearly a year. All the photos taken on the left are before any injection. The photos on the right were taken a *year* after her previous injection.

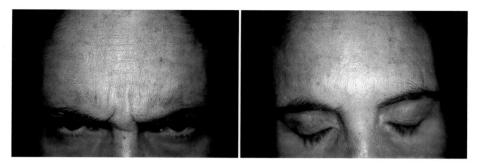

Figures 83 and 84: Frowning.

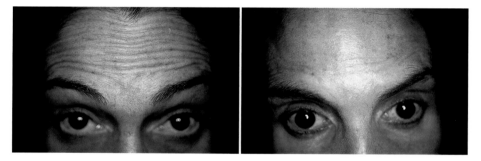

Figures 85 and 86: Raising eyebrows.

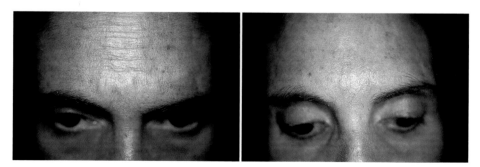

Figures 87 and 88: At rest. This patient was able to achieve long-term results with her Botox injections. She also achieved a long-term Botox browlift. The patient is five years *older* in the pictures on the right.

Figures 89–92: The patients below achieved long-term results from their injections.

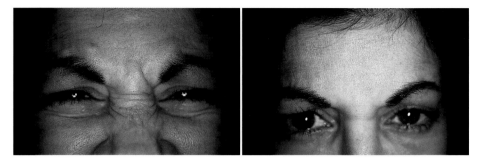

Figures 89 and 90: Frowning. Original photo and seven months after her last injection.

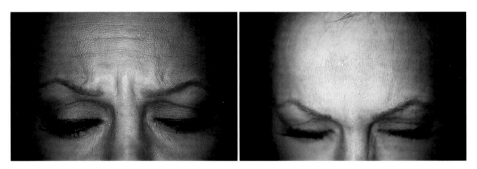

Figures 91 and 92: Frowning. Original photo and nine months after her last injection.

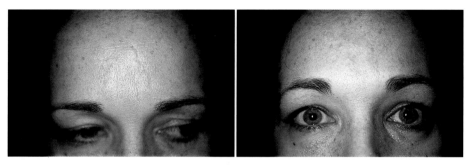

Figures 93 and 94: This patient's forehead and brow were treated for five years with Botox. Over these years, the patient has noticed that a forehead scar that she has had since the age of sixteen has faded away. The patient is five years older on the right!

Figures 95 and 96: This patient in her thirties requested lower eyelid surgery to remove the "bags" beneath her lower eyelids. The "bags" were actually a roll of muscle along her entire lower eyelid, which smoothed out nicely after her Botox injection. She is smiling in both pictures.

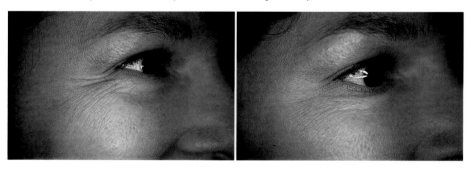

Figures 97 and 98: This patient in her forties was primarily concerned about her strong frown lines. She received Botox injections to her frown and forehead areas. Although improved, some frown lines, which were then injected with a filler material, remained.

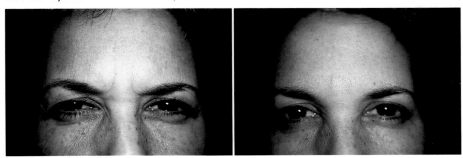

Frowning before and after both injections. She could not have received this degree of improvement after injection of either Botox or filler material alone.

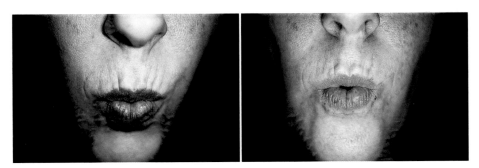

Figures 99 and 100: In this patient, Botox has been used to weaken the "smoker's lines" around the mouth. She was asked to whistle in both photos.

Figures 101–104: The patients on this page had poor outcomes from surgical procedures that were later treated with Botox injections.

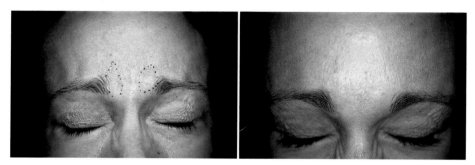

Figures 101 and 102: This patient had an endoscopic browlift that left her still able to frown and with two dents in her brow. Botox was used to weaken the frown muscles and fat was injected into the outlined indented areas.

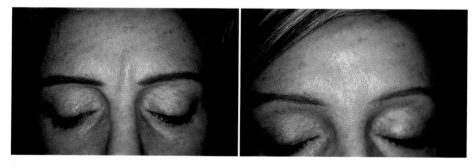

Figures 103 and 104: A patient with more severe linear indentations that were also treated with Botox followed by fat injections.

no working muscle will be left. So using this analogy, you might thinking that it would be possible to repeatedly inject Botox into a muscle for two years and it would not ever work again. But in reality, that doesn't happen. That is why you have to actually observe, follow, and pay attention to your patients.

So far, we've been talking only about the frowning muscles. That is where long-term weakening first becomes apparent in my patients. That's because these are the muscles that I weaken the most. I have never had long-term atrophy in the muscles of the lower face or neck. That's because, to achieve a good cosmetic effect, these muscles should be only slightly weakened. I have occasionally seen long-term effects in the forehead and less often in the crow's feet area. Again, that is because the forehead and crow's feet are only partially weakened. These muscles have real functions other than wrinkling your skin. The forehead muscles have to hold the eyebrows up. The crow's feet muscle is responsible for closing your eye and holding your lower eyelid up. Totally paralyzing either of these muscles would be irresponsible for the average patient.

Timing Is Everything

So does everyone who has Botox injections over several years get some atrophy of the frowning muscles? The answer is no. And I don't just mean for the people with exaggerated facial motion. I mean the average patient who has been treated over a long period of time. Just having multiple Botox injections over many years is not enough to produce the desired atrophy.

Timing is the key variable. If you are the kind of person who allows your Botox and your resulting weakness to completely wear off before your next injection, it is unlikely that you will ever develop long-term effects. That is because, as in the broken-arm example, you are allowing that arm to regain its full strength. Then, with the next injection you're starting all over again. The clock has been reset.

But if you're the kind of patient who wants very little motion, and you return closer to three months rather than six or seven months after your prior injection, you most likely will develop some long-term weakening of your frowning muscles.

So what about the middle-of-the-road patient who comes back every four to five months? This is the majority of my practice. Most of these patients will develop some weakening of the frowning muscles, but it usually takes several years. I have seen weakening of these muscles in patients who are injected every three months after only a year and a half.

While timing is the most important variable, dosage is also a key. Most of my patients desire some long-term weakening of these muscles. Depending on the interval between their injections, some start to see it within two years and others do not start to see it until after four or five years. But timing isn't the only variable. Very often, I will see patients who are just starting to experience some long-term weakening of the frowning muscles. They will lament that although their frowning area looks good, they are in the office to have their chins or crow's feet areas done since it doesn't seem to last as long in these areas. And they are right. It doesn't last as long in these areas because there are so many viable nerve endings right next to the muscle fibers that they reconnect to them more quickly, resulting in full motion. But usually, there's a little motion in the frown area, so I like to inject all the areas at once in the patient. The question is how large a dose should I put in this muscle? Almost always, I put in the full dose that has worked well for that patient. Most of my patients would rather go for the possibility of a long-term result. To them, it's worth a little extra pain at the time of injection. I also think that this is why in some other offices, long-term results are not often seen. I have heard other injectors say that they greatly reduce the dose for the frowning muscles on these occasions, since the patients cannot tell the difference anyway. That way they are saving themselves a couple of dollars but denying their patients a chance for long-term results. And then after a few months go by and the patient is due to be injected again, the frowning muscles will be relatively stronger compared to the other muscles, since they didn't have a full dose at the prior treatment session. I don't "short" my patients on their Botox doses.

Resistance Is Futile

One concern about using Botox over and over in patients is the development of resistance. That is why some doctors refuse to give touch-up injections and insist that patients only be seen no sooner than three months between injections. Three months is also the interval for injections approved by the FDA. Theoretically, when a long protein like Botox is introduced into a patient repetitively, it can spur the body to produce antibodies to the Botox, rendering it ineffective. According to most models, this is more likely to happen when high doses are used and when the interval between injections is short. The question is how high a dose and how short an interval is needed to develop resistance. For instance, patients with cerebral palsy who have much higher doses of Botox injected still very rarely develop resistance. Cerebral palsy patients often have the very large muscles in their legs injected to reduce muscle spasms. This may spare them surgery, which actually cuts the tendons of these overactive muscles.

I have been doing small, touch-up injections in my patients for eleven years. I do not routinely divide my doses and give them to patients in stages (except for patients at an extremely high risk for developing eyelid droop). But if I feel an area on patients has been underinjected, I do not hesitate to improve their appearance by injecting a drop or two here or there. I have never seen complete resistance to Botox in any of my patients. In a handful of patients, I've noticed a slight diminution of effect over several years. But I have never seen someone not respond to Botox. If someone were to develop immunity to Botox, there is an alternative. Myobloc has been available for over a year. Myobloc is botulinum toxin type B. The areas on these two different proteins that develop antibodies are different. So if someone develops antibodies to type A, the person does not a necessarily have antibodies to type B. Even if a patient eventually develops full resistance, the person would still have an alternative treatment.

Line-Free Is Not the Goal

The greatest misunderstanding about Botox is the idea that when used properly, it totally eliminates a person's expression. Another misconception was seen in a cartoon that recently appeared in a New York magazine. In the cartoon, a woman who is apparently as stiff as a board is being carried under a man's arm. The caption reads something to the effect of "Honey, aren't you overdoing the Botox a bit?" Of course, this is exactly the opposite of what Botox does. Botox doesn't make your muscles stiff, it relaxes them. When a muscle is completely relaxed then that muscle is paralyzed. Botox has a bad name primarily when it is overdone.

Certain muscles of the face do nothing but wrinkle the skin above them. When these creases become etched in the skin so that they are present even when the face is at rest, patients often seek help. The creases are there for a few reasons. One, that muscle has creased that patch of skin thousands of times a day for many years. This beat up the skin so much that the creases are there even when the muscle isn't trying to crease the skin. Second, over time the skin becomes thinner and less elastic and therefore more prone to wrinkling. Third, over the years, the relative strength of these muscles become stronger than their surrounding tissues. So much so that even when the face is at rest, there is some resting tone in these muscles pulling the skin to create a crease. Using Botox affects two of these reasons. It stops the muscle from pulling even when it is at rest, and weakens the muscle so much that when contracting it does not contract and beat up the skin as much as it normally would.

The key to using Botox effectively is not only deciding where the patient's problem areas are, and which muscles or parts of muscles to inject, but also deciding how much to weaken different parts of different muscles. In my mind there is a happy medium. In the best-case scenario you are giving up a tiny bit of expression for a lot fewer lines. In the vast majority of people this is an excellent trade. Trying to trade no expression for no lines is not a good trade. The ideal situation exists when patients have no lines at rest but are able to crease and move their face when animated. This must be kept in mind when a patient repeatedly requests long-term results. Long-term results can be more readily achieved when a muscle is completely or nearly completely paralyzed. But who cares if you are successful long-term if the patient does not look good trying to get there? I do not let the patient's desire for long-term results negatively affect the cosmetic result that I can achieve in the present with Botox.

The woman in Figs. 89 and 90 is in her thirties and had only been injected for a little over two years. Despite that relatively short time, she definitely had some atrophy of her frowning muscles. If she did not have any atrophy, she would be able to frown just as strongly in Fig. 90 as she can in Fig. 89. Without atrophy, after seven months, her Botox should have completely worn off. The woman in Figs. 91 and 92 had used Botox for nearly four years when the photo on the right was taken. Even after eleven months, she barely has any motion. Both of these patients were reinjected with their normal full dose.

Typical Patient After Ten Years

At medical meetings, I'm often asked about the long-term effects of Botox on my patients. Other physicians are rightfully concerned about the possibility of total irreversible muscle atrophy of the facial muscles of expression. Especially since some of these muscles actually have an important function. This has never happened in any of my patients. What has happened is something that my patients like. These patients, of course, develop long-term results but never irreversible atrophy. While some patients come and go over the years, some are very loyal. A few years ago, when the popularity of Botox skyrocketed, I saw an old patient of mine whom I had not seen for well over a year. We exchanged pleasantries, and I examined her face. I asked her when her last Botox injection was. She said she wasn't sure, why don't I just look at her chart.

I then corrected her, telling her I did not mean her last injection given by me, but her last injection. She looked at me strangely and said she would never go anywhere else, that I had given her her last injection. Despite the fact that it was over a year from her prior injection, she still looked pretty good. In fact, the motion of her muscles was not as strong as it was several years ago before I began injecting her. This is something that I see more and more of.

The typical patient whom I've been injecting for about ten years usually needs to be injected only about every year to year and a half. As these patients have already achieved a long-term result, I do decrease their dose a bit. I don't do it just to save on Botox. I do it because with the muscles weakened, giving these patients their previous full dose would make them appear overly paralyzed. But while coming to the office less often, having fewer injections, and spending less money is something that most patients like, it's not what they like the most.

The best thing about these patients is their prolonged honeymoon period. When patients are just starting out with injections, they can look a tad overdone for the first four weeks, then look pretty good for another four weeks, then look outstanding for a month or two. It is in this last phase that, I feel, the best results are seen. This is after the skin has been rested, the muscles are weakened but not paralyzed, the patient has virtually no wrinkles at rest, and has a natural expression when animated. Shortly after this phase, the lines start to come back a little bit heavier, and then they are present even at rest. It is this honeymoon phase in the middle where patients look their best. But early on, patients cycle through peaks and valleys of less animation, honeymoon phase, more lines, and repeat. The best part about long-term results is that this honeymoon phase is greatly extended. The patients' expression and appearance no longer go through peaks and valleys but long plateaus of a rested, smooth, natural appearance.

This honeymoon phase is also something I try to get patients into for a big event. For instance, sometimes patients will tell me that their child is getting married on such and such a date and so they want a Botox appointment one week before. I will tell them not to do it so soon beforehand. What if they get a bruise? What if they beat the odds and get a droopy eyelid? Even if they did not have one of these unlikely events befall them, why not have their Botox look its best and most natural? Depending on how long I have been injecting them and how long their results last, I usually recommend they have their injection four to ten weeks before the event. The same scheduling applies to actors and actresses with a film role to prepare for. During the honeymoon phase, performers have the perfect balance of fewer lines and natural expression. Throw in the fact that immediately before the "honeymoon" the skin has been on a "vacation" from being creased repeatedly by its muscles and you have fans wondering "How does she look so great?"

The patient in Figs. 83 through 88 had a nice long-term result from her prior injections in both her frowning muscles and forehead. Even her Botox browlift is evident after a year. What she liked the best about her long-term result was her lengthy honeymoon phase. For most of the prior year she had no lines when at rest. In fact, she was so happy with the honeymoon phase she was in that we mutually decided not to inject her at that visit—she wanted to ride out her honeymoon phase as long as she could.

8

THE FOUNTAIN OF YOUTH

~~~~~~~~~~~~~~~~~~~~~~~~~~
~~~~~~~~~~~~~~~~~~~~~~~~~~

We have seen how Botox can work. It's great for removing fine to moderate lines around the face and neck. Botox can also change certain facial characteristics from unflattering to attractive. But does it really make you look younger? That's not a simple question to answer. And the question really needs to be broken down over the short-term and long-term.

Over the short-term, Botox may help you to appear a little bit younger but not very much. What it really does is help you look *better*. There are a lot of different characteristics about people's appearance that makes us think of them as younger or older. Of course it all boils down to younger or older than what? The obvious answer is their actual age. This is where a little of my personal philosophy kicks in. Basically, I don't care how old someone is. That is true in my personal life as well as my professional life. I think it's just about the least important thing that I can find out about someone.

First, let's be clear about what sort of age we are talking about. There is your physiological age. This factors in how well you take care of yourself, how much you exercise, what shape your heart and lungs are in. Then there is your mental age. I know some people in their forties who act and think as though they are in their twenties. I know some people in their thirties who act as though they are seventy. I have known people in their nineties who were incredibly mentally sharp. Certain relatives of mine appear to be senile in their early fifties. Then there's something ghastly called your actuarial age. This was devised by people who work for insurance companies to try to determine how many years someone has left. They factor in all sorts of things from your occupation, to whether you are right or left-handed (left-handed people live an average of nine years less than right-handed people), your health habits, your family history, and where you live. They then give you a number. This number does not represent how many years you've lived but how many you probably have left until your death. But what most people talk about is their chronological age. In other words, their age depending strictly upon the day they were born.

You may say that this year indicates certain shared experiences other people born close to that year may have. But I've had shared experiences with people decades older or younger than myself. People mature at different ages. In spite of this, people's attitudes, accomplishments, and appearance are often indexed to their chronological age. When the gossip columns or glossy magazines say that an actress of sixty-five and an actress of twenty-five look good, they often are saying two different things. They're saying that the twenty-five-year-old is beautiful. They are implying that the sixty-five-year-old looks good for her age. It's the "for her age" part that I resent. It shouldn't matter. If you want to look good, want to look good. If someone looks good for her age, does that phrase imply that she doesn't really look that good?

When someone is chronicled in *People* magazine or the newspaper, after her name usually comes her age. Why? Who cares? Are people being written about because they are thirty-eight years old? Or are they being written about because they are newsworthy because of something they did? Are we supposed to be jealous or happy that someone achieved some level of success, or fame, or notoriety at a chronological age younger or older than we are now? I don't care. In my personal life, I haven't asked anyone how old the person is for several years.

My professional life is a different story. Although I am a plastic surgeon, I like to think that I kept some of the qualities of the good old-fashioned country doctor. What people often call antiaging medicine but which I think is more appropriately termed age-management medicine has a lot of parallels with plastic surgery. I've attended quite a few lectures and courses about this new subspecialty. And although I do not dispense vitamins or hormones or other serious age-management medications for my patients, I do gently prompt them to keep up with things to protect their general health. For instance, at different ages, it is recommended that someone receive a mammogram, a prostate exam, a colonoscopy, and so on. When it comes to protecting your health with general screening measures, age is important. When it comes to discussing with my patients the risks involved with surgery and anesthesia, age is important. Chronological age is not as important as someone's overall health, but it is still a factor. That's why I ask every one of my patients how old they are. It is not because I am sizing them up and trying to determine if they look good or bad for their age.

Patients often ask me at what age I recommend they get a facelift. That is an impossible question to answer. When I determine what procedures I would do to improve someone's appearance, I do not think about their age at all. You may think this a bit disingenuous, but it is not. You may think that if I have a young lady in her mid-twenties in my office with sun damage and heavy wrinkles across her upper face I would be more likely to treat her with Botox. My response would be, more likely than what? Anyone who fit that description would be a good candidate for Botox. Then you might ask, how about the seventy-five-year-old patient with wrinkles but lots of excess skin sagging across the face? My response would be that I do not care how old she is. Anyone with a lot of sagging skin would only be a marginal candidate for Botox. It depends on what they have on their face and what tools I have to fix it.

In America, we are definitely age obsessed. And more than a little too wrapped up in what we see in the mirror.

That being said, does Botox really make you look younger? Person-
ally, in the short-term, I think that's unusual. I think you can look
dramatically better, but if I had to guess I would think that you would
look about the same age as before we started. What would be dramatically different is if you appeared haggard, beat up, and run through the
mill. This is something Botox can dramatically change. But I am a professional. Maybe your friends, acquaintances, and you yourself may think
you look younger. Especially you. *The Wrinkle Report,* based on a poll
by Louis Hans and Associates, was published in the 1990s. It surveyed
baby boomers to see what they thought about aging. Three out of four
boomers said they look younger than their age. Eight out of ten said
they had fewer signs of facial aging than other people their age.

They also tend to look at some things through rose-colored glasses.
It is statistically impossible for such a high percentage of people to look
younger than their age. If it were true, then how someone looked for
that age would need to be adjusted more youthfully. If most people of
a certain chronological age look a certain way, then that is how the
average person looks for that age. On the whole, it is a bit of a mass
delusion.

If that's the case, why do I consider Botox an antiaging procedure?
Because I think, over time, Botox is the single best antiaging therapy
there is. Period. Botox is different from all other procedures aimed at
eliminating lines and wrinkles. Other procedures like collagen injections,
fat injections, laser resurfacing, chemical peels, and surgery all try to
correct the symptom. And the symptom is what we see, the wrinkling of
the skin. None of these treatments attempts to correct the root cause of
the problem. Of the lines and wrinkles that we see on the face, most are
caused by the action of muscles below the skin. Sure, sun exposure,
aging and thinning of the skin, and gravity contribute. As of now, we
don't have any antigravity or age-reversing machines or treatments. But
we do have an antiaging muscle drug. If you can prevent these muscles
from crinkling your skin thousands of times a day over many years, you
will look a lot better than if that were not the case.

Even in patients with severe, deep lines the results can be amazing.

Very often these patients have only a modest improvement when they start out using Botox. But since the skin is such a vital, living organ, it can heal itself and repair itself over years when external stresses such as strong muscles, smoking, and the sun have been removed. These patients often see their best results over a period of years. Looking back at my patients over many years, I see some amazing results. Very often, since Botox has improved their appearance so much, my patients start to clean up their act in other areas as well. Since their faces started to look better, many of my patients have also stopped smoking and stopped abusing their skin with the sun. These are both things that my patients knew were bad for them for many years. I do not scold my patients who engage in these practices. I gently remind them that it is not good for them. I do not treat my patients like children. Sometimes, the little nudge that Botox gives them is all they need to start living lives that are healthier for their skin (and the rest of them too).

Even if someone doesn't change bad habits, Botox works wonders over years. Look at my patient in Figs. 83 through 88. We're not going to talk about long-term results again. But just look at her appearance. Both sets of photos were taken without any Botox effect on board. If someone told you that one set of photos was taken five years before the other set, which set would you guess were taken of the patient at the younger age? I think it's pretty obvious. But the photos on the right show the patient five years *later* than the photos on the left. Unfortunately, this patient did not change any of her habits. She was still a sun person and a heavy smoker. All the result that you see was simply due to regular Botox injections over several years. Just imagine how much more improvement she could have attained if her skin were healthy.

What we have talked about so far were purely objective results. Results that you can see just by looking at the skin in photographs of patients. But something else happens to my patients who have Botox injections. Something that you cannot see just by looking at them. I have had countless patients tell me that since they were injected, they just feel better. They feel better about their families, jobs, spouses, and life.

But Botox does not have any psychological effects. What are these patients talking about?

I think some of it may be due to a little biofeedback. When patients
are angry, they make angry faces. After many years, this pattern is deeply
ingrained in all of us. Right now, if you are alone, I want you to try a
little exercise. Make the meanest, most threatening face that you can and
at the same time try to talk in your sweetest baby-talk voice possible.
Then try it the other way around. Say something in the most sinister,
nasty voice possible (try Linda Blair in *The Exorcist*) with a kind smile
on your face. Next to impossible. Even if you can do it, it takes a great
deal of concentration. Over time I think certain behaviors become hard-
wired to certain facial expressions as well as body language. Being unable
to make an angry face in some patients actually helps to prevent them
from becoming very angry. Granted, it's a little like putting the cart
before the horse, but I think that is the way it works for some people.

Everyone likes looking better. At the end of a hard day, it just gives
you one less thing to worry about. And vanity is not the nasty word you
think it is. People are vain. Everyone is vain. To my mind it is just a
question of degree. If people were not vain, they would all walk around
wearing a potato sack over their heads for clothing and a simple pair of
shoes. Well, maybe not a real potato sack, but a more comfortable potato
sack. Maybe a potato sack with some pockets. Maybe a potato sack with
long sleeves for cold weather. If it weren't for vanity, there would be no
point in trying to dress differently from anyone else. There would probably be one standard shoe. A shoe that after years of cobblers searching
for perfection was simply the most comfortable shoe that could be made.
No one would care what it looked like. At least not without some degree
of vanity. If it were not for vanity, there would be no such thing as
makeup or hair styles. We would all get our hair cut enough to keep it
out of our eyes. We would all be walking around with bowl haircuts.
Have you ever worn makeup? Case closed. We are all vain. Vain people
like to look good. That is another reason Botox makes us feel good.

Another reason for feeling good after Botox is the one that I think
has the biggest effect for most people. Sure, how we feel about ourselves

deals with our own thoughts, fears, and yes, appearance. But people are social animals. Even the grumpiest people who say that they always want to be left alone need human contact. That's why the worst punishment you can get in a maximum-security prison is being separated from the rest of the prisoners. Yes, it's true, human beings would rather live their lives among a pack of known murderers than spend it alone. How we feel depends a lot (probably too much) on how these other people deal with us. It has to do with what they do, what they say, and even the expression on their face when they are talking to us. Not to mention their body language. What happens is if you seem less angry, less nasty, less put out, less haggard, people are kinder, brighter, and nicer to you. Over the course of a day, weeks, or months if people who are important in your life and even people who are not are consistently gentler and kinder to you, it will have a positive effect on your sense of well-being. Even the Grinch was won over by the inhabitants of Whoville.

On a more scientific note, self-esteem is very important to one's sense of self. There is obviously quite a boost to anyone's self-esteem when the person looks better in the mirror. Especially when what has changed is something that had been bothering them for many years. And whether we like it or not, in contemporary society there are definite benefits to physical attractiveness. People go out of their way to be nicer and to be closer to people who are physically attractive. It is not fair, but it is the way people are. Changing your appearance sets off a complex set of emotional triggers.

Are we too wrapped up by what we see in the mirror? I think so. Although I *am* a plastic surgeon, I think that there is probably too much plastic surgery going on. Overall, I think it is done too often, too early, and too aggressively. There is a fine line between wanting to look really good and insecurity about your appearance. Which is why I never use the word *need* when I am discussing a procedure with a patient. If the time comes when patients ask me if they *need* Botox or plastic surgery and I say yes, it is time to retire. People have enough insecurities and problems in their life without a plastic surgeon telling them they need to have something done.

9

THE FUTURE

~~~~~~~~~~~~~~~~~~~~~~
~~~~~~~~~~~~~~~~~~~~~~

The Botox revolution began over a decade ago and now seems to be reaching its peak—or is it? Despite the fact that 1.6 million people had Botox injections in 2001, that number is sure to go much higher. All those brave people had off-label usage of Botox. Since the FDA approval is relatively narrow compared to the scope of what Botox can actually do, most people that I am injecting now and will inject in the future will also be injected off-label. But being able to market this drug to the general public as an aesthetic medication, even for just the area between the brows, means that the 1.6 million number is sure to skyrocket. While Botox has been sort of old hat among trendsetters in America's biggest cities, now everyone will know about it. The problem is, it will also produce an increase in demand for physicians injecting it. That means more and more physicians who did not have aesthetics emphasized during their residency training will be injecting Botox. It also means there will probably be more and more poor injecting and Botox horror stories in the tabloids.

Looking into my crystal ball, I see some highs and lows for Botox in the immediate and distant future. With all the hype and press coverage and marketing, the buzz on Botox will be very positive and use will increase. This is sure to be followed by a backlash. Just as there will be new patients, there will be new injectors. Lots of them. Some may not be so honest about how many Botox injections they have done. Some will not have had good (or any) training. This will lead to patients being overly weakened. Truly paralyzed patients will start to pop up at work, at the mall, and on the street. As with any cosmetic treatment, there tends to be a little more guilt and cattiness when things go wrong. One truly spectacular failure lingers in the collective public consciousness more than a thousand successes. When I'm at a party and I first meet someone, what do you think the person wants to talk about? Jocelyn Wildenstein (the cat lady), Michael Jackson, and Joan Rivers.

Allergan's study, which included 263 patients and was presented at the American Academy of Dermatology meeting in March 2000, introduced work done by multiple injectors. The authors of this paper were the Carruthers; Nick Lowe, M.D., and M. A. Menter, M.D. The incidence of eyelid droop in the patients who had well-trained injectors was over 5 percent. How often do you think it will happen when practically every Tom, Dick, and Harry with a medical license (or nurse's license) begins to inject it? Although if you go to a talented injector, Botox can help you look great, do not assume that the handsome stranger you saw in the hallway was winking at you; he just may not be able to open his eye.

The other backlash is unfortunately something that may happen partially because of this book. I expect it will cause Botox injections to areas of the lower face and neck to increase. After all, in these areas you can achieve outstanding results. They are also the trickiest areas to inject and are most definitely not for the Botox novice. Injecting these muscles takes a great deal of finesse, anatomical knowlege, and patience. (I have a high touch-up rate for these areas—especially the first time around.) After the initial upswing of injecting in these areas, I can predict what you will start to hear: "It does not really work around the mouth." "Someone was drooling for months after an injection." "A friend of a friend of a friend couldn't smile or drink from a straw."

Despite these horror stories, which I am quite sure you will hear, Botox is going to be around for a long time. In the hands of a talented injector administered to a properly selected patient, the results are just too good.

So is there a challenger who might knock Botox off its throne? Myobloc has been approved for use for neck spasms in America since December 2000. Like Botox, it is a strain of the chemical made by the botulism bacteria. There are eight different strains that have been identified. Botox is botulinum toxin type A and Myobloc is botulinum toxin type B. Both are large protein molecules. Both prevent the nerve from communicating with its muscle. But how they accomplish that is slightly different. Botox breaks up a protein that the nerve needs to send its signal to the muscle. Myobloc does that too, although it breaks up a different protein. So while on a large scale their mechanism of action is the same, on a molecular scale, their actions are different.

There are different parts of these long proteins that the body could potentially react to and make antibodies against. This would render either medication ineffective. These areas are different on the different proteins. For that reason, it is extremely unlikely that anyone who might become immune to Botox would also be immune to Myobloc. And vice versa. So how does Myobloc stack up against the champion, Botox?

Besides working with Allergan, I have also served as an advisory board member to Elan. As of this writing, I have been using Myobloc in my practice for one year. In April 2002, I was asked to give a presentation on Myobloc for my plastic surgery society. There are several interesting differences between how Myobloc and Botox work clinically. The main advantage to the patient of using Myobloc is that it works much more quickly than Botox. When I inject patients with Botox, I tell them not to look for any change for at least two days, which is usually the earliest that someone will see the effect of the medication. Quite often, it takes five to seven days before the patient sees the final result. Occasionally, the patient will see a change immediately after the injection. This change is not due to the action of the medication, which is very slow-acting. Initially, the lines may look better because of the saltwater that's injected along with the Botox. This acts as a temporary filler material, making fine lines appear smoother. The second reason is if the injection was done properly, the Botox was delivered directly into the muscle. These muscles are very small and fragile and the trauma alone of having a needle and some medication injected into them may make it tough for them to work at full strength for a few hours—as if this tiny muscle has a charley horse. Myobloc usually shows some results within six hours. The final result typically takes two to three days. But if someone had an important event that evening, a Myobloc injection would be able to help the person look better by that deadline.

The other advantage that Myobloc has is for the physician, especially someone who does not have a very busy practice when it comes to weakening muscles for cosmetic effect. According to the manufacturer, once a vial of Botox has been mixed, it should be used within four hours. Most people realize you can keep it a bit longer than that. Since I do Botox every day that I'm in my office, the Botox I use is always fresh. But that's not true for a lot of injectors. In America, the lion's share of injections is done by a relatively few injectors who are very busy. Then there are a great many injectors who inject Botox only occasionally. These occasional injectors sometimes use Botox that may be several weeks old. I have been surprised by the number of people who tell me that they use Botox that is a month old and say that it is almost as good. I think that is one of the reasons why occasionally I'll see patients in my office who had been injected elsewhere and were told when they complained that they didn't have much of a result that they were immune to Botox. I think that sometimes patients are injected with an old, weak solution. Myobloc is an advantage for these injectors. It comes premixed and has a shelf life of at least nine months. This makes it advantageous for the injector who only occasionally does Botox or who is just starting out in practice and doesn't have very many patients.

So this sounds pretty good so far, and frankly, I think there will always be some good uses for Myobloc. But it has some disadvantages as well when compared to Botox. It comes ready to inject, but Myobloc is slightly more acidic than Botox. For this reason, it hurts and burns a bit more upon injection. It may be possible, in the future, for this solution to be neutralized a bit so that it does not burn so much. But those studies have not been done yet. Currently, neutralizing Myobloc may decrease its effectiveness, and for that reason I have not neutralized it. I have injected myself with both Botox and Myobloc. And while Myobloc definitely hurt a bit more, it was not "night and day" more. But there absolutely was an increase in burning immediately upon and after injection.

The other current drawback to Myobloc is in its duration. Even with its being slightly more painful, I think some of my more stoic patients would prefer Myobloc because it works a bit faster than Botox. But what patients don't seem to be willing to compromise on is duration of effect. When injecting Myobloc, I used gradually increasing doses to see if I could get it to last as long or longer than Botox. Initially, it lasted about half as long as Botox. At higher doses, its effect was still a bit shorter than that of Botox but at least comparable. In fact, several of the photographs in this book were taken after patients had Myobloc injections. Figs. 33 and 34 of the woman's crow's feet were Myobloc photos. My own photos in Figs. 47 through 50 were also taken before and after Myobloc injection. The first patient I ever injected with Myobloc was myself. Before I used it on any of my patients, I wanted to be able to honestly tell them about the difference in pain and effect that I thought they might experience. If I was willing to try it on my patients, I certainly should have been willing to try it on myself. The smile line photos of Figs. 61 through 64 were taken before and two months after Myobloc. This was one of the better long-term results I had with Myobloc, but this patient thought that by three months all of her results were gone. The chin photos of Figs. 69 through 74 were also taken after Myobloc. This patient had been a longtime Botox patient. Initially she was quite pleased with the results despite the slight increase in pain. But she was unhappy with the longevity of her result compared to what she achieved with Botox. The lip photos from Figs. 99 and 100 were also done with Myobloc. All the other photos in the book were taken after Botox injection.

Currently, my Myobloc patients have a duration of results about three-quarters as long as my Botox patients after they first began to have injections. I cannot tell you if Myobloc patients' results will increase in duration of action because I haven't been using it that long. What I will tell you is that patients I injected with Myobloc who had never been treated with Botox were extremely happy with their results. Patients who had had Botox injections previously were primarily unhappy with the shorter duration of action. They weren't crazy about the increased pain either after becoming accustomed to Botox.

So where does Myobloc fit in? Well, possibly with even higher doses, the longevity of Myobloc may be increased. I did not go extremely high with my doses, since I felt it left my patients looking a little too weakened. It may be feasible for Botox and Myobloc to be injected together. Since they work by different mechanisms, this could potentially give some added benefit. For myself, I always plan to keep a vial of Myobloc handy. If the patient has a big event that day or the next, I would use Myobloc. There are even some examples when the decreased duration of effect is a big advantage.

I discussed Botox and laser resurfacing earlier. Most physicians agree that the two when combined have excellent results. The Botox keeps the skin from crinkling while the skin is in its healing phase after the resurfacing. This helps to diminish recurrent lines from forming during the healing. When the skin's new surface is forming, you do not want it to be wrinkled by the muscles beneath it. The result is smoother skin. But Botox lasts for several months. Therefore, most physicians inject Botox only in the typical areas that I've discussed earlier in this book. But if these areas will look better if they don't move during the healing, why wouldn't this apply to every area of the face? Last year, I had a patient who had severe acne when she was a teenager. She was now in her thirties and her skin had been clear for many years. We discussed her options and decided to do laser resurfacing of her face. Since she did not have much in the way of dynamic lines around her face, she had not been receiving Botox injections. Her resurfacing was not for wrinkles but for acne scarring. I wanted her face to heal with the best result possible. After discussing it with her beforehand, as soon as I was finished doing her laser resurfacing, I injected almost every muscle in her face with Myobloc at a low dose. Myobloc was the perfect medication for this particular patient. Since Myobloc worked so quickly, the patient would not be moving and wrinkling her face during her early healing phase. If I had injected her with Botox, she would have been wrinkling her face for three to five days after her procedure. The other problem would have been that although her skin would have been healed (although a bit red) at two weeks, she would still have looked very strange. No one looks good with a completely paralyzed face. This would have lasted for at least a few months, so she would have been either a shut-in or someone who was stared at all that time. But with low doses of Myobloc, her face was paralyzed early and yet her paralysis began to wear off after only two to three weeks. This was the best of both worlds. She was motionless during her healing phase and yet she regained motion just as her skin was finally healed.

Another good area for Myobloc will be during scar revision, when it is imperative that no tension be placed across the newly forming scar. That way, the scar will be as thin as possible. The problem is, scars are not always in a good area for patients to be paralyzed. Because of that, Myobloc would be a good choice, because during the early stages of wound healing the scar would not be subjected to tension or additional forces from muscular action across the skin. And the patient would not have to endure months of looking strange due to paralysis in an area of the face that needs to move. I have used Myobloc for that purpose in my office. A few months ago, I directly excised a portion of the frowning muscles beneath a patient's eyebrows. This was done through a very small incision right through the eyebrow itself. At the same time, I also injected fat into the rather severe frown lines this patient had. I thought that permanently weakening her frowning muscles as well as placing filler material into her deep wrinkles was the ideal procedure for her. But I also wanted the small incision inside her eyebrows to heal without a noticeable scar. And I wanted her fat injections to live and last as long as possible. I knew that keeping this area from moving would help to accomplish both of those goals. So I injected this patient with Myobloc during the procedure when I was looking directly at the muscles I was injecting through the small incision in her eyebrows. Due to the local anesthesia, she couldn't wiggle her eyebrows for a few hours after the procedure anyway. Once that was gone, the Myobloc kicked in and prevented her from having motion across either of her incisions or the lines into which her fat had been placed. The quick onset of Myobloc's action was the key here.

One disadvantage of using Myobloc could be the price. One unit of one drug does not equal one unit of the other. Myobloc was initially priced so that fifty units cost the same as one unit of Botox. From looking at their comparable uses in the neck, that is what most people thought the proper ratio might be. Unfortunately, that turned out not to be the case. My dose of Myobloc differed depending on the area of the face but it was frequently between 125 to 150 units for the typical unit dose of Botox for the same area. So an equivalent amount of Myobloc could cost three times as much as Botox. It remains to be seen what the company will do about the pricing of this drug.

I am more comfortable and can get better results from a strictly cosmetic standpoint with Botox. But I have only been using Myobloc for a year in about thirty patients. Contrast this with injecting Botox for eleven years in many thousands of patients. Right now, if I have a difficult problem needing a lot of precision, Botox is my choice. If someone's face is fairly asymmetrical, if I need to raise one brow more than the other, or in any other finesse-type injection, Botox is my only choice.

Another drug that has not arrived yet in America is named Dysport. Dysport, like Botox, is botulinum toxin type A. Dysport has been available and widely used in Europe for cosmetic purposes for many years. As yet, it has not been FDA-approved for any use in human beings in America. Consequently, I have never injected Dysport. However, the company that manufactures it is in the process of applying for their FDA approval. That is not a quick process. It is estimated that it may take two to three years for that approval to come through. Although they are both botulinum toxin type A, there are some differences between Dysport and Botox. Besides the protein molecules that actually do the work, there are other proteins included in both preparations. The amount of these proteins is different between the two solutions. Even in countries where both products have been widely available, there is some disagreement as to how many units of Dysport equal how many units of Botox. The units are not equivalent.

The future for Botox is bright indeed. I see it being used by more and more people. That will happen partly from marketing and partly from envy. As discussed before, baby boomers are very competitive, especially when it comes to appearance. They are obsessed with looking good for their age. When their neighbors, friends, and coworkers start looking better through proper use of Botox, it will raise the bar in their eyes. Even if they do not really like the idea, some will feel compelled to use Botox just to keep up with whom they see as the competition, namely everyone. That is unfortunate. Ideal usage of Botox should help you to feel better about yourself.

I also hope to see Botox doses going down in search of a more natural look, with a balance between weakness and strength in the face. Overall, the face of a paralyzed person looks bad. Small areas look better. Generally, strong faces look better than weak ones. Younger faces are stronger, not weaker faces. That is why many people have used facial exercisers for years. Strong muscles help to hold the face up. They help to increase the circulation to the skin. In a perfect world, people would be using highly specific muscle stimulators to strengthen muscles that help to support and hold the skin up and very precise low-dose Botox injections to weaken muscles that pull things down and crinkle the skin heavily. I have been asked many times about the seeming contradictions of Botox and muscle stimulators having beneficial cosmetic effects. My response is, although at an immediate level they do perform completely opposite functions, when muscles for each are targeted correctly, their effects are synergistic.

10

JUST THE FAQS

WILL A BOTOX INJECTION HURT?

Yes, although not as much as a bee sting or going to the dentist. But Botox does involve several small injections made with a needle. Ice will be used beforehand so that the pinching sensation is dulled.

HOW LONG WILL IT TAKE?

For the initial visit, discussion, examination, and injection about half an hour. Once the injections begin, it's all over in about half a minute if you are just doing frown lines, or four to five minutes if you're doing multiple areas.

HOW LONG WILL IT LAST?

For most people starting out, the injections work really well for about three months and then give diminishing returns for about another three to four months. Every patient is different. Also, some areas tend to have longer-lasting results than other areas of the face and neck. Typically, the frowning area lasts the longest, whereas areas around the mouth last the least amount of time.

IS THERE AN ADVANTAGE TO STARTING YOUNGER? OR A DISADVANTAGE?

Usually it is to the patient's advantage to start younger. That way you can prevent the muscles beneath your skin from wrinkling the skin so deeply that permanent deep lines are formed. But I am not an advocate of prophylactic Botox injection. In other words, if you're very happy about the way you look and do not want anything changed, I would tell you not to get Botox injections just because they may help you in the future. Helping your skin to resist aging forces is, to my mind, a pleasant side effect of your Botox injections and should not be the main purpose of your treatment.

WILL I FEEL NUMB?

No, you will not. Some patients describe a strange sensation when muscles that they are trying to move have been weakened. Sometimes they describe this as feeling numb. But if you were to touch these areas, you would certainly feel it as you do normally. Botox does not affect your sense of touch.

WHAT WILL I LOOK LIKE AFTER MY INJECTION?

The overwhelming majority of patients walk out of my treatment room with just a few small red dots at the areas that have been injected. These marks typically take fifteen minutes to go away. After that, there is no sign to tell anyone that you have had an injection. Rarely, someone may develop a small bruise. This is something that can be easily concealed with makeup.

HOW SOON CAN I WEAR MAKEUP AFTERWARD?

I allow my patients to apply makeup as soon as they leave the treatment room.

WILL I HAVE PROBLEMS PUTTING MAKEUP ON?

No. Despite what you may have heard, your skin's sensation is completely intact.

CAN I RECEIVE A FACIAL OR MASSAGE AFTERWARD?

Not for the first two hours. After two hours, you can do anything you wish.

CAN I FLY AFTER A BOTOX INJECTION?

Flying is permitted two hours after injection.

WHAT AREAS CAN BOTOX WORK ON?

Over the years, I have injected every single muscle in the face as well as some muscles in the neck, chest, forearms, and hands. The best areas for cosmetic uses of Botox are the frown lines between the eyes, worry lines across the forehead, crow's feet lines around the outer eye area, to raise or lower or change the shape of the eyebrows, the smile lines between the nose and the mouth, the little vertical lines coming up from your upper lip and down from your lower lip, wrinkles between the lower lip and chin, and the neck.

HOW MUCH DOES IT COST?

This depends on how many areas you will have treated as well as where you live. In general, the cost ranges from about $500 to $1,500.

HOW CAN I FIND SOMEONE NEAR ME TO INJECT BOTOX?

The best way is a referral from a friend who is happy with her injector. You should also think she looks good after her injection. Other ways are to contact the American Academy of Dermatology (888-462-DDRM) or the American Society for Aesthetic Plastic Surgery (888-ASAPS-11). You can also look at the Web site for thebotoxbook or findabotoxexpert. The physicians listed here have at least heard me speak or watched me perform injections on people.

WILL IT WORK FOR MY SKIN?

That depends on how deep your lines are and the condition of your skin. While age also factors in, it is not the single most important factor. How healthy your skin is and how deep your lines are already are more important. Sun exposure, cigarette smoking, and heavy drinking all damage your skin's ability to resist wrinkling and to bounce back after your Botox injection.

CAN I GET BOTULISM FROM AN INJECTION?

The amount of Botox given during a typical cosmetic injection is too small to give a healthy patient a botulismlike illness.

I'VE BEEN TOLD THAT I CAN'T READ A BOOK
AFTER BOTOX INJECTIONS. IS THIS TRUE?

Every physician has his own instructions for patients after a Botox injection. My instructions are very simple. My patients are told not to engage in any heavy lifting, straining, or other activity that would raise their heart rate for two hours after their injection. I tell my patients that they are permitted to lie down, to read, and to pursue all normal activity. They are also allowed to bend to pick something up. However, I prefer it if they bend more at their knees and less at their waist.

WHAT ARE THE RISKS INVOLVED WITH THE BOTOX INJECTION?

The number-one risk that most patients are afraid of is a droopy eyelid after injection. Among my own patients, this happens less than one-half of 1 percent of the time. But there are risk factors that can predispose you to having this reaction. During your examination, these should be looked for and discussed. Some patients may get a bruise after their injection. Some patients also complain of a headache after injection.

IS THERE ANY WAY TO PREVENT A BRUISE OR HEADACHE?

Yes, there are certain things patients can do beforehand to reduce the risk of these unwanted events. First, avoid aspirin, Advil, Motrin, Aleeve, Nuprin, and products similar to and containing these substances before your injection. Sometimes these medications can affect you for as long as two weeks after you've taken them. Being calm and breathing deeply during your injection can also help to limit headache after injection. An experienced injector can also avoid triggering headaches in most patients.

CAN BOTOX INJECTIONS REPLACE A FACELIFT OR BROWLIFT?

A facelift does many different things that Botox cannot do. A browlift is also different from Botox, though Botox can do many of the things that a browlift does. So for the patient whose brows are just a little droopy, yes, Botox can usually lift the brows a bit and help you to put off that surgery.

CAN A BROWLIFT TAKE THE PLACE OF BOTOX INJECTIONS?

Sometimes. However, the way that most surgical browlifts are done today, Botox is usually a helpful adjunct and can actually improve and possibly prolong the effects of your surgery.

IS THERE ANYONE WHO SHOULD NOT HAVE BOTOX INJECTIONS?

Yes. Anyone who has a neuromuscular disorder should not have Botox injections. Some of the more common disorders are myasthenia gravis and Lambert-Eaton syndrome. Also, patients who were on aminoglycoside antibiotics should not have Botox injections. I also do not inject women who are pregnant, who are nursing, or who are trying to become pregnant.

IS IT TRUE THAT BOTOX LASTS LONGER AND LONGER THE MORE YOU DO IT?

For most people, yes. What is important is the interval between Botox injections. If you allow your motion to come back to 100 percent before getting another injection you probably will not see any long-term lengthening of effect.

HOW LONG DOES IT TAKE TO WORK?

Most patients start to see some effect at two to three days after injection. For the final result, it often takes five to seven days.

IF I GET THE DREADED DROOPY EYELID, WHEN DOES IT HAPPEN AND HOW LONG DOES IT LAST?

Typically, the droopy eyelid appears about five days after injection. In my practice, it usually lasts for one and a half weeks. Patients will start with a slight amount of droopiness at the beginning. Very often they do not even notice it themselves, but it is pointed out by someone else. This minor annoyance then becomes more noticeable for a few days and then gradually gets better day by day until it is gone. The whole cycle lasts about ten days for most people. While it is going on, the droop often appears worse at the end of the day and is less noticeable in the morning.

CAN I GET BOTOX INJECTIONS IF I HAVE A COLD?

Yes. Your cold will not affect the results of your injections, nor will your injections have an adverse effect on your cold. But I also tell my patients that if they are ill for whatever reason, why put themselves through a medical procedure that is unnecessary and purely cosmetic in nature? I prefer to have them wait until they are feeling better.

I HAVE HEARD OF SOMEONE NOT BEING ABLE TO SWALLOW OR SPEAK AFTER AN INJECTION; IS THIS POSSIBLE?

I have never seen nor heard of this happening after a Botox injection for cosmetic purposes. You must realize that Botox is used in much higher doses in deeper muscles of the neck for certain medical conditions. Under those circumstances, this unwanted complication could be possible.

WILL I LOOKED PARALYZED AFTER MY INJECTION?

Not if you go to a good injector. In my opinion, Botox should almost never be used to completely paralyze a muscle. The cosmetic results are much better if selected muscles are only partially weakened, leaving the patient with a very natural result.

CAN I DRINK AFTER MY INJECTION?

Again, since drinking increases the circulation throughout your face, I prefer my patients not to consume alcohol for two hours after their injection.

CAN I GO OUT IN THE SUN AFTER MY BOTOX INJECTION?

Sun exposure does not adversely affect the Botox itself. However, I can't advocate sun exposure for any of my patients.

CAN I USE BOTOX IF I AM USING RETIN-A, GLYCOLIC ACID, OR OTHER HARSH FACIAL PRODUCTS?

Yes. These products do not have a negative effect on your Botox injections. With proper application, they may actually help your skin to look as good as possible after your injection.